DEAFNESS IN CHILDHOOD

EDITED WITH A PREFACE BY

DEAFNESS IN CHILDHOOD

FREEMAN McCONNELL, Ph.D. AND PAUL H. WARD, M.D.

Vanderbilt University Press

DEDICATED TO

William   Wesley   Wilkerson,   Jr.,   M.D.

1897-1961

This study was supported in part by a grant from the Children's Bureau, United States Department of Health, Education, and Welfare.

PREFACE

THE twenty chapters of this book were presented as papers at the National Symposium on Deafness in Childhood at Vanderbilt University on May 5 and 6, 1966. Sponsored by the Bill Wilkerson Hearing and Speech Center and the Division of Otolaryngology of the Vanderbilt University School of Medicine, this symposium marked the tenth anniversary of the groundbreaking ceremony for the Bill Wilkerson Hearing and Speech Center. This center has served as a clinical and teaching laboratory in affiliation with Vanderbilt University since its founding and has always shown a major concern for the needs of the young deaf child. The symposium brought together more than four hundred distinguished guests from the fields of audiology, otolaryngology, and education of the deaf from throughout the United States who shared this concern.

The introductory chapter by Sir Terence Cawthorne is the First Wilkerson Memorial Lecture, a featured presentation of the Symposium, given in honor of the late Dr. W. W. Wilkerson, whose far-sighted vision and dedication to the needs of speech- and hearing-handicapped individuals combined to produce a unique, statewide speech and hearing program in Tennessee. Dr. Wilkerson was firmly committed to the principle that service, teaching, and research must move forward in close interrelation if the problems besetting society in the management of those with communication disorders are to be effectively solved. He was also convinced that audiology and medicine should develop a close working relationship that would result, not only in the most effective care of the speech and hearing handicapped person, but would also enhance the progress of these disciplines themselves.

From his convictions emerged the Bill Wilkerson Hearing and Speech Center, named by the Board of Directors in 1952 in honor of Dr. Wilkerson's son who lost his life in World War II.

It was the aim of the symposium to reflect the philosophy that the needs of the deaf child require the integrated efforts of both medical and nonmedical specialists. It is hoped that bringing together in printed form these papers by eminent leaders in the fields of otology, audiology, and education of the deaf will result in a valuable addition to the literature on the problems of childhood deafness. Editing has been kept to a minimum in an effort to convey the generally informal communicative spirit of the symposium. The concluding chapter was the address delivered by Sir Terence as an after-dinner talk given at the symposium banquet and is included to provide a note of entertainment for the reader—a diversion as refreshing and enjoyable as it was for the participants in the symposium.

The symposium and the resulting publication would not have been possible without the generous support of the United States Children's Bureau, Department of Health, Education and Welfare, and the Tennessee Hearing and Speech Foundation. Grateful acknowledgment is owed both of these agencies. Acknowledgment is also expressed to a host of others, including members of the Symposium Program Committee, the staff members of the Bill Wilkerson Hearing and Speech Center and of the Division of Otolaryngology at Vanderbilt University, each of the centers of the Tennessee Hearing and Speech Foundation, and to the many others in the University Center whose cooperation was proffered so willingly.

Freeman McConnell
Paul H. Ward

CONTENTS

THE AUTHORS

RUTH E. BENDER, PH.D., Associate Director, Cleveland Hearing and Speech Center, and Assistant Clinical Professor, Western Reserve University, Cleveland, Ohio

La VONNE BERGSTROM, M.D., Resident Physician, Division of Otolaryngology, University of Colorado School of Medicine, Denver, Colorado

JOHN BORDLEY, M. D., Professor of Otology, Johns Hopkins University School of Medicine, Baltimore, Maryland

PATRICK E. BROOKHAUSER, M.D., Fellow, General Surgery, The Johns Hopkins University School of Medicine, Baltimore, Maryland

KENNETH S. BROWN, M.D., Surgeon, United States Public Health Service, and Investigator, Human Genetics Branch, National Institute for Dental Research, Bethesda, Maryland

RAYMOND CARHART, PH.D., Professor of Audiology, Auditory Research Laboratory, Northwestern University, Evanston, Illinois

LEO E. CONNOR, ED.D., Superintendent, Lexington School for the Deaf; and Lecturer, Teachers College, Columbia University, New York City.

MRS. MARION P. DOWNS, M.A., Director of Clinical Audiology, University of Colorado School of Medicine, Denver, Colorado

JOHN H. GAETH, PH.D., Professor of Audiology, School of Medicine, Wayne State University, Detroit, Michigan

ROBERT GOLDSTEIN, PH.D., Professor of Communicative Disorders, Department of Communicative Disorders and Department of Rehabilitation Medicine, School of Medicine, University of Wisconsin, Madison Wisconsin. Formerly Director, Division of Audiology and Speech Pathology, The Jewish Hospital of St. Louis; Associate Professor of Audiology, Washington University, St. Louis, Missouri

VICTOR GOODHILL, M.D., Professor of Surgery in Residence (Otology), University of California, Los Angeles, California

FREDERICK R. GUILFORD, Clinical Professor of Otolaryngology, Baylor University School of Medicine, Houston, Texas

JANET HARDY, M.D., Associate Professor of Pediatrics, The Johns Hopkins University School of Medicine, Baltimore, Maryland

WILLIAM G. HARDY, PH.D., Associate Professor of Laryngology and Otology, The Johns Hopkins University School of Medicine, Baltimore, Maryland

JOSEPH E. HAWKINS, JR., PH.D., Clinical Professor of Physiological Acoustics, Kresge Hearing Research Institute, University of Michigan School of Medicine, Ann Arbor, Michigan

WILLIAM G. HEMENWAY, M.D., Associate Professor and Head, Division of Otolaryngology, University of Colorado Medical Center, Denver, Colorado

JAMES JERGER, PH.D., Director of Research, Houston Speech and Hearing Center; Research Associate Professor of Audiology, Baylor University College of Medicine, Houston, Texas

JOHN R. LINDSAY, M.D., Professor and Chairman, Division of Otolaryngology, University of Chicago, Chicago, Illinois

EDGAR L. LOWELL, PH.D., Administrator, John Tracy Clinic, Los Angeles, California

HARRIET MANTELL, M.D., Chief Pediatrician, Lehigh Valley Society for Crippled Children and Adults, Muhlenberg Medical Center, Bethlehem, Pennsylvania. Formerly Chief Pediatrician, Multiple Handicapped Clinic, Children's Mercy Hospital, Kansas City, Missouri.

HELMER R. MYKLEBUST, ED.D., Director, Institute for Language Disorders and Professor, Language Pathology and Psychology, Northwestern University, Evanston, Illinois

RALPH NAUNTON, M.D., Professor of Otolaryngology, University of Chicago, Chicago, Illinois

HAYES A. NEWBY, PH.D., Professor and Director, Division of Speech Pathology and Audiology, Stanford University School of Medicine, Palo Alto, California

ARTHUR I. NEYHUS, PH.D., Associate Professor, Deaf Education and Guidance, Northwestern University, Evanston, Illinois

HAROLD SCHUKNECHT, M.D., Professor of Otology and Laryngology, Harvard Medical School; Chief of Otolaryngology, Massachusetts Eye and Ear Infirmary, Boston, Massachusetts

GEORGE E. SHAMBAUGH, JR., M.D., Professor of Otolaryngology, Emeritus, Northwestern University School of Medicine, Evanston, Illinois

CATHERINE, SMITH, PH.D., Research Associate and Professor of Otolaryngology, Washington University School of Medicine, St. Louis, Missouri

THE FIRST WILKERSON MEMORIAL LECTURER

SIR TERENCE CAWTHORNE, F.R.C.S., England; Hon. M.D., Uppsala; Hon. LL.D., Syracuse; Hon. F.R.C.S., Ireland

AURAL SURGEON, National Hospital for Nervous Diseases, Queen Square, London; Consulting Adviser in Otolaryngology to the Ministry of Health, England; Director of the Otological Research Unit, Medical Research Council, National Hospital for Nervous Diseases, Queen Square, London; Honorary Consulting Surgeon, Diseases of the Ear, Nose, and Throat, King's College Hospital, London.

CHAIRMEN OF THE MEETINGS

LOUIS M. DICARLO, PH.D., Hammond Professor, Audiology and Speech Pathology, Syracuse University; and Associate Clinical Professor of Otolaryngology, Upstate New York University Medical School, Syracuse, New York

THEODORE WALSH, M.D., Professor and Chairman, Department of Otolaryngology, Washington University School of Medicine, St. Louis, Missouri

THE PROGRAM COMMITTEE
NATIONAL SYMPOSIUM ON DEAFNESS IN CHILDHOOD

Coordinators

Freeman McConnell and Paul Ward

The Committee

RAYMOND CARHART, PH.D., Professor of Audiology, Auditory Research Laboratory, Northwestern University, Evanston, Illinois

AMOS CHRISTIE, M.D., Professor and Chairman, Department of Pediatrics, Vanderbilt University School of Medicine; Member of Executive Committee, Bill Wilkerson Hearing and Speech Center, Nashville, Tennessee

WILLIAM G. HARDY, PH.D., Director, Hearing and Speech Center, The Johns Hopkins Medical Institutions, Baltimore, Maryland

DONALD A. HARRINGTON, PH.D., Consultant, Speech and Hearing, Children's Bureau, Department of Health, Education and Welfare, Washington, D. C.

MRS. KATHRYN HORTON, M.S., Coordinator of Student Training, Bill Wilkerson Hearing and Speech Center; Instructor in Speech Pathology, Vanderbilt University School of Medicine and Secretary, Tennessee Hearing and Speech Foundation, Nashville, Tennessee

R. H. KAMPMEIER, M.D., Director of Continuing Education, Vanderbilt University School of Medicine, Nashville, Tennessee

WILLIAM G. KENNON, M.D., Assistant Clinical Professor of Otolaryngology, Vanderbilt University School of Medicine, Nashville, Tennessee

JOHN R. LINDSAY, M.D., Professor and Chairman, Division of Otolaryngology, University of Chicago, Chicago, Illinois

FREEMAN McCONNELL, PH.D., Director, The Bill Wilkerson Hearing and Speech Center; Professor and Chairman, Division of Audiology and Speech Pathology, Vanderbilt University School of Medicine, Nashville, Tennessee

JAY SANDERS, PH.D., Director of Research, Bill Wilkerson Hearing and Speech Center; Associate Professor of Audiology, Vanderbilt University School of Medicine, Nashville, Tennessee

HAROLD SCHUKNECHT, M.D., Professor of Otology and Laryngology,

Harvard Medical School; Chief of Otolaryngology, Massachusetts Eye and Ear Infirmary, Boston, Massachusetts

GEORGE E. SHAMBAUGH, JR., M.D., Professor of Otolaryngology, Emeritus, Northwestern University School of Medicine, Evanston, Illinois

RICHARD W. STREAM, PH.D., Chief Audiologist, Bill Wilkerson Hearing and Speech Center; Assistant Professor of Audiology, Vanderbilt University School of Medicine. Nashville, Tennessee

W. O. VAUGHAN, M.D., Associate Clinical Professor of Pediatrics, Vanderbilt University School of Medicine, Nashville, Tennessee

PAUL H. WARD, M.D., Associate Professor and Chairman, Division of Otolaryngology, Vanderbilt University School of Medicine; Member of Board of Directors, Bill Wilkerson Hearing and Speech Center,

PART I

THE PROBLEM

The First Wilkerson Memorial Lecture:
CHILDREN WITH DEFECTIVE HEARING

I DEEPLY appreciate the honor which the Trustees of the Foundation have paid me by inviting me to give the First Wilkerson Memorial Lecture, and I am grateful to the United States Children's Bureau and the Tennessee Hearing and Speech Foundation for making my visit possible.

I was glad to learn that deafness in children would be an acceptable subject for this lecture because this has compelled me to crystallize my thoughts and call upon my past experience in the investigation, care, and management of deaf children.

At the end of the war I became Chief Aurist to the Education Department of the London County Council and this post carried with it the otological care and supervision of some five hundred children. At that time, just after the war, many of the children had been evacuated to special schools throughout the country and much reorganization was necessary before they could be brought back to London. The time seemed ripe for the introduction of units for partially deaf children under the care of special teachers of the deaf in ordinary schools. Four schools were chosen and the scheme has been very successful, and after a short term in a special unit many of the pupils have been graduated to classes of normal-hearing children.

The late Miss Edith Whetnall took over this post from me in 1947, and I have always been glad to have played some small part in arousing her interest and enthusiasm in this fascinating subject. Only last year the Nuffield Speech and Hearing Centre was opened in London under her direction, and it is very sad that she did not live long enough to see it in full working order.

3

But it will be a memorial to remind us all of the great work that she did for deaf children.

I first met the Ewings of Manchester before the War, and I always enjoyed the visits that I paid to them. Indeed, I am very grateful to Sir Alexander and the late Lady Irene Ewing for the generous and openhearted way in which they shared their experience with me and for what they taught me. Then, towards the end of the war, the Medical Research Council established an Educational Treatment of Deafness Committee, under the Chairmanship of Sir Frederick Bartlett, on which I served and which included Sir Alexander and the late Lady Irene Ewing, teachers of the deaf, inspectors of education, otologists and physicists. Through the Committee I learned much of the current thinking of those whose interest was the care and education of deaf children.

My personal knowledge of institutions on the North American Continent is limited to the Central Institute for the Deaf, the John Tracy Clinic of Los Angeles, the clinic set up by the late Dr. Wishart at the Toronto Sick Children's Hospital, the Clinic at Syracuse University inspired by my great friend Dr. Gordon Hoople, and now I can add the Bill Wilkerson Hearing and Speech Center. The great work carried out in each of these clinics is an inspiration to all, and there are many other such clinics in the United States which have achieved international fame.

Like everyone who has at any time been interested in deaf children, I have certain views about the many problems presented by these children, and I will during the course of my discourse try to bring these out; for it is my firm belief and one which now seems to be shared by many others that the management and care of deaf children is a combined operation calling for the whole-hearted co-operation of many disciplines—one that does not delegate to any discipline the automatic right to leadership. I am quite sure that the *primus inter pares* principle is the right one, just as the sharing and pooling of knowledge as between disciplines is another.

All these disciplines, including teaching, physics, bioengineering, psychology, physiology, otology and the testing of hearing, may be gathered together under one umbrella—that of audiology. I well remember Gunnar Holmgren of Sweden organized two very successful conferences on audiology and I had the honor of being Secretary for the Second Conference in Stockholm when he was President. Now we have an International Congress of

Audiology; the last meeting, and a very successful one it was too, was held in Copenhagen, Denmark, in 1964 under the presidency of Professor Ewertson. It was a very enjoyable and fruitful congress, but I could not help feeling that the audience would have been able to understand the contributions better if each speaker had addressed himself to the audience at large in words and language more readily appreciated by a general than by a special audience. In any congress that embraces many disciplines there is always the temptation for each speaker to address his remarks to his fellows rather than to the audience at large.

I believe that if all these disciplines were more accustomed to explaining to their colleagues in other disciplines in a hearing and speech center what they meant it would help towards a better understanding of these often difficult and highly technical problems.

Hearing, Speech and Language

The greatest attraction at the Zoo in London is the chimpanzees' tea-party held every summer afternoon at 4:00 o'clock.

Before a delighted audience, four of these apes, dressed up as children and seated at a tea table, are served by their keeper with tea, bread and butter and cakes, and the odd piece of fruit on the side. Their general behavior (apart from occasional and much appreciated lapses) is well up to human standard, including their appreciation of applause with a tendency to play up to their audience in the hope of earning even more applause. They can obviously hear, see, smell, touch and taste; but they cannot be taught to speak. Like so many other animals, they can communicate their emotions vocally and by grimaces, but they cannot put their thoughts, such as they are, into words.

The ability to speak and the precious gift of language is peculiar to man, and it is this wonderful faculty which, by enabling him to speak and to listen to ideas and thoughts, has made him supreme in the kingdom of living creatures. Certainly, it is not man's ability to run, to swim, to climb, to exert his strength, nor yet the sharpness of his senses that has earned him this superiority. If one could imagine an Olympic contest for all living creatures, man would not gain even a Bronze Medal in any event. But if there were a contest for oratory, man would be the only entrant, for only he can voice his thoughts. It is true that certain birds, notably parrots, can imitate human speech sounds, but they have no appreciation of language.

Clearly, it is the comparative size and the quality of man's brain that has enabled him to develop, out of cries, grunts, squeals, song and babbling, speech and eventually language.

My friend and colleague, Dr. Macdonald Critchley, in his Monograph on "The Language of Gesture" has suggested that gesture as a form of communication may have evolved at the same time as speech, and he gives several instances of certain primitive groups who use gesture instead of speech, as in the Australian aborigines and the earlier North American Indians. I shall refer to this again presently.

One of the loveliest events of which every parent of a normal child is an entranced witness is the gradual change from babbling (which is the formless and meaningless exercise of the organs of speech) into words, the first of which may well emerge by the age of a year. By two years old, short sentences may be expected, with a vocabulary of at least 50 words, by the age of five, 2000 words. The basic mechanism whereby this miracle occurs is threefold. Sound is picked up by the ear and carried to the temporal lobe of the brain which, after much practice, sends appropriate messages via the motor speech area to the vocal organs. These again, after much practice, are able to repeat what they hear or to reply to a question. Thus, speech and eventually language develop. In this connection, it is interesting to note that Dutch and Danish observers have been able to detect an intonation typical of the infant's native language in its babbling some time before any word has been voiced.

By far the commonest cause of any delay in the development of speech is an imperfection in the organ of hearing which prevents the infant from hearing properly the words and sentences addressed to him by the members of his family. Depending upon the severity of the hearing defect, his speech will be delayed, distorted, or absent.

It is generally agreed that one in every thousand children is born with such a severe hearing defect that he will never learn to speak by the normal way of imitating what he hears. Another and possibly larger group may have a partial defect in hearing sufficient to delay or to impair the development of properly pronounced words.

Severe or total deafness which does not develop until after language has been learned, though tragic, is not such a handicap as deafness at birth which prevents the normal development of language.

Historical Background

It is a pleasure to acknowledge my indebtedness to Dr. Ruth Bender from whose book *The Conquest of Deafness* I have learned so much of the history of deafness in children.

From the writings of the past it seems likely that deaf mutism was as common in the earlier days of civilization as it is now. It was mentioned in the Bible and by the early Greek and Latin writers, and it will be interesting to trace the fate of the deaf mute throughout the ages. But in doing so we must appreciate that such deafening diseases as meningitis and severe bilateral suppurative otitis media were much commoner before antibiotics and sulphonamides were available than they are now. I can remember only too well before the advent of these miraculous drugs how common severe deafness and its attendant speech disorders were when bilateral suppurative ear disease attacked an infant before it had learned to speak.

The Age of Miracles

The plight of the deaf-mute was clearly appreciated in Biblical times and in the Roman era, for the Hebrew Law differentiated between those who were deaf and dumb and were denied legal rights and those who were deaf only. This was expressed later in the Justinian Code of Laws in which those born deaf and dumb were, like children and lunatics, without legal rights or obligations; on the other hand, those who became deaf after acquiring language were deemed capable of managing their own affairs. As we shall see later, this denial of legal rights to those born deaf and dumb was the strong stimulus that led to teaching of the deaf.

We are given a vivid picture of the miraculous cure of a deaf and dumb young man by Our Lord in the Gospel according to St. Mark. This was the first of the Gospels, written about 100 A.D., and was full of action rather than doctrine.

Starting with the baptism of Jesus Christ by St. John in the River Jordan, the disciples were drawn from the fisherman on the shores of the Sea of Galilee. Then a series of miraculous cures was related. The mother-in-law of Simon was cured of a fever, a leper was cleansed, two unclean spirits (presumably madness) were driven out, the recently deceased young daughter of a ruler of the Synagogue was raised from the dead, a woman who had suffered from an issue of blood for twelve years was cured, a man who was sick of the palsy walked again, a deaf and dumb man spoke again after his ears and his tongue had been touched by Our Lord, a blind man had his sight restored, and an epileptic was cured of his fits.

All these miraculous cures were of disorders common enough even in those days. But then they were not amenable to any cure or special management, and, as we learn from the Gospel according to St. Mark, nothing short of a miracle could help.

Apart from a short reference in 685 A.D. by the English chronicler the Venerable Bede to the restoration of speech to a deaf and dumb man by the Bishop of Hagulstad (who later became St. John of Beverly on the North East coast of England and is the Patron Saint of the deaf and dumb), nothing is recorded in this field until after the Renaissance.

The Age of Teaching

This age extended from the Renaissance till the last quarter of the nineteenth century. Most of the teachers were priests in holy orders as was usual even into the twentieth century. It was also an age in which many teachers of the deaf guarded the secret of their system so carefully that the method died with them, and it was an age in which teaching the oral method clashed with teaching by signing, finger-spelling, and writing. It is only fair to say at this point that these ages are not strictly separated, and it may well be that the contest between the oralists and the signers has not yet ceased. There may be good reasons for this as I shall explain later on.

That remarkable and universal genius Leonardo da Vinci mentions the deaf and dumb and draws attention to their ability to lip-read. Then Rudolf Agricola from Groningen in Northern Holland mentions a deaf-mute who had learned to express his thoughts in writing. But it is Pedro Ponce de Leon of Spain who is regarded as the first teacher of deaf-mutes. Born of a noble family in 1520, he became a monk in the Monastery of San Salvador where he worked and taught until his death in 1584.

His pupils came from wealthy and famous families among whom were two deaf and dumb sons of the Constable of Castile. The elder Francisco was heir to a Marquisate with accompanying property and fortune, and through Ponce de Leon's teaching he acquired enough language to enable him to claim his birthright. All records of his teaching were lost in a fire in the Monastery library, but it is interesting to speculate why it should have been in Spain rather than Italy that the teaching of deaf-mutes was established.

It is true that Spain was at the height of her civilization and had added much of the New World to her kingdom. It is of particular interest that the first entry into North America by the Spanish was a Juan Ponce de Leon who occupied and named Florida, and claimed it for Spain. Perhaps he was a relative of the monk? Perhaps he came into contact with the North American Indians who because of the multiplicity of languages (more than 65) had developed a sign language whereby strange tribes could communicate. They also relied on communication by gesture when hunting demanded silence. Such a sign language could have been brought back to Spain and used as a basis of communication between deaf-mutes.

Ponce de Leon was followed by Bonet in Spain who wrote the first book in 1620 on sign language making use of a one-handed alphabet. He made no reference to Ponce de Leon, although he taught a deaf relative of the children taught by Ponce de Leon. In his book, Bonet makes the trenchant remark that for the deaf mute to understand what is said to him by the motions of the lips and tongue no teaching is necessary. Though we may be excused from agreeing with this entirely, it is only fair to say that many of the most accomplished lip readers appear to have been self-taught. I have always been impressed by the relationship between natural intelligence and the ability to learn lip reading. I will refer to this again later on.

Later on in the 1620s Prince Charles of England was on a visit to Philip IV of Spain and was interested in a young deaf Spanish lord, a pupil of Bonet's, who was an expert lip reader. Sir Kenelm Digby, who was in Prince Charles' suite, remarked on how the young deaf Lord had been able to hold a conversation with anyone provided he could see their lips.

After the publication of Bonet's book, more interest was shown in sign language than in lip reading. Anthony Densing (1660), Professor of Medicine at Groningen, wrote an essay on the deaf-dumb, expressing the view that because of the close connection between the nerves of hearing and the nerves of the tongue, damage to one might easily implicate the other. Shortly before this, Felix Platter of Basle published a book on anatomy and one of the plates showed the nerves leading from the tongue to the region of the ear. Platter, in common with other anatomists of his time, thought these were all branches of the same nerve leading to and from the brain. A century later we hear of Samuel Heinecke of Germany who decided to use taste as well as sight and touch in teaching deaf children. In his method, water on the tongue indicated the vowel A, sweet water the vowel E, wormwood the Vowel O, vinegar the vowel I and olive oil for U. To us this sounds far fetched and even absurd, but there is some reasoning behind it when we recall that the chorda tympani nerve which takes taste sensation from the tongue to the brain actually passes through the middle ear and in between the ossicles.

The reason for this is that the outer and the middle ear are developed from the primitive gill clefts and arches which form part of the human embryo in the course of development. These are a relic of the gills of our fishy ancestors, and the nerve of taste in fish is situated in the gills to enable the fish to recognize the taste of the water constantly being pumped through its gills. This is how, for instance, a salmon recognizes its home river on its way back from the ocean—by means of the chorda tympani nerve in the gills.

Those of us who operate for otosclerotic deafness find that the chorda tympani nerve is very much in the way as it threads through between the incus and the malleus, and it may have to be displaced or sometimes even cut. In the days of Heinicke and Platter the difference between sensory and motor nerves was not appreciated, so it is no wonder that the chorda tympani nerve suggested an intimate nervous connection between the tongue and the ear which accounted for the association between hearing and speech. Dalgarno of Scotland published a manual alphabet in 1661, and Amman of Switzerland who settled in Amsterdam in 1690 published his famous work *Surdus Loquens* which told of his method of teaching the deaf and dumb to talk and to hear with their eyes, for he re-introduced lip reading and his method found favor, particularly in Germany.

One who has been described as the greatest teacher of all was Pereira who settled in Bordeaux in 1741 after being driven out of Spain (he was a Jew) into Portugal. It has been said that his interest in deaf mutes was aroused by a beloved sister who was deaf and dumb. He achieved great success in France as a teacher and came to the notice of the Royal Family and was even elected a Fellow of the Royal Society of London. Unfortunately, like so many before and after him, he was most secretive ·about his methods and each of his pupils had to promise not to reveal the secrets of his successful teaching. Unfortunately, he failed to pass on either his methods or his talent to his family, so that after his death his son was unable to keep his father's practice going, nor were his widow and daughters any more successful.

The Abbe de l'Epee is perhaps the best known of all teachers of the deaf. Born at Versailles in 1741, he entered the priesthood, and a chance meeting with deaf twin sisters on a parochial visit aroused his interest and he taught them to write—but not to speak.

He learned Spanish in order to read Bonet's book. He took into his house, which soon became a school for deaf children, poor and rich alike. King Louis XVI gave him the revenues from a suppressed convent which enabled him to extend his work and to establish a state school for all who needed the special help he and his staff were able to offer.

In 1776 he published a book on sign language as the method of choice for the instruction of deaf mutes. He believed that the signs made by the deaf with their hands were the basis for a universal language whereby the deaf throughout the world could communicate. This observation is supported by Macdonald Critchley in his monograph on the *Language of Gesture* who observes that sign language as used by deaf mutes has a great deal in common with the sign language as used by the Aborigines of Australia and the North American Indians.

In 1936, at a service in St. Pauls' Cathedral, London, attended by deaf mutes from fourteen different countries, all the delegates were able to follow the sermon translated into sign language for their benefit. On the other hand, lip reading has to be learned for each language, so that deaf mutes from, say, Italy, Egypt, and England would be unable to converse with one another except by means of signs.

Of course, the major objection to sign language is that only those learn it who are compelled to do so; that is to say, the deaf themselves and their relatives, teachers, and spiritual advisers, will be able to understand it. Thus the deaf can only take their part in the life of the community if they can learn lip reading. Another objection to signing is that it does not encourage vocalization.

But to get back to L'Abbe de l'Epee, he attracted attention from the rulers of many other countries, including Austria and Russia, and he trained teachers from many lands.

When he died in 1789, one of his pupils, the Abbe Sicard, succeeded him. The Abbe Sicard managed to survive the perils of the French Revolution, and the school flourished under his care. Another pupil of de l'Epee was the Dutchman, Guyot, who founded the Groningen Institution for Deaf-mutes in 1790. His methods were based on the sign language he had learned from de l'Epee; he also encouraged his pupils to speak.

In Scotland, Thomas Braidwood, a teacher born in 1715, became interested in teaching deaf mutes as the result of teaching the deaf child of a wealthy Glasgow merchant. One thing led to another and Braidwood's method, though secret, consisted basically in teaching his pupils lip reading and writing. He attracted much attention. Even the great Samuel Johnson, who visited Braidwood in Edinburgh, commenting on what he saw, said, "It was pleasing to see one of the most desperate of human calamities capable of so much help."

In 1783, Braidwood moved to Hackney near London where he was joined by a nephew, who, after Thomas Braidwood's death in 1806 published a two-volume *Instruction of the Deaf and Dumb by the Oral Method.*

A grandson of Thomas Braidwood emigrated to the United States where he started a deaf school, but his intemperate habits soon led to disaster.

In the last quarter of the eighteenth century interest in the deaf and dumb was aroused in the United States, and Charles Green of Boston visited England and was trained in the Braidwood School.

In 1810 the Reverend John Stanford discovered several deaf children in the New York almshouse and established a school for them. This led in 1818 to the opening of the New York Institution for the Deaf and Dumb with sixty pupils.

Then the Reverend Thomas Hopkins Gallaudet, after he was graduated from Yale in law in 1805, took up the study of theology and began his ministry at Andover, Massachusetts, in 1814. Soon after this he became interested in Alice Cogswell, a deaf child aged nine, whose father, Dr. Cogswell, was his neighbor, and started to teach her. Dr. Cogswell was reluctant to follow the fashion then of sending his daughter to Europe for special education, and on inquiring into the incidence of deaf mutism he found that there were eighty in the State of Connecticut alone.

Dr. Cogswell therefore put it to his influential friends that there was an urgent need for education of the deaf in their state. It was agreed to send the Reverend Gallaudet over to England to study the oral method of the Braidwoods. When he arrived in England, he confided to the Braidwood family that he wished to study their oral method and the signing method which held favor in France, under the Abbe Sicard. This did not suit the Braidwoods and, meeting the Abbe Sicard who was on a lecture demonstration tour in London, he explained his difficulty and was invited to Paris where he trained with Sicard. When he returned to the United States, Gallaudet was accompanied by a young French pupil-teacher who was deaf. Almost a year later in 1817 the American Asylum for the Deaf was opened in Hartford with seven pupils, and a year later the pupils numbered forty. The oral method was abandoned, communication being by signs, finger spelling, and writing.

On the continent of Europe, with the exception of France, lip reading was the preferred method of teaching.

Once again, Scotland provided one of the immortal names in the annals of deaf teachers and of communication in the person of Alexander Graham Bell. His father, Alexander Melville Bell, emigrated to Canada in 1871, hoping that the climate would save their son Graham who was threatened with pulmonary tuberculosis. His two brothers had already died from this disease. The father, Alexander Melville Bell, was already known in Boston where he had lectured the previous year on visible speech and elocution. In 1872 Alexander Graham Bell opened in Boston a training school for teachers of the deaf based on the oral method, but the opposition of the silent school was such that he changed it to a school of Vocal Physiology or Elocution.

Mabel Hubbard, a deaf young woman who had been to Germany to learn the oral method, came to Bell's school to improve her speech. They fell in love and for five years Bell labored to evolve an electrical machine which would transmit speech. He succeeded in this and was granted a patent on what turned out to be the first telephone. Alexander Graham Bell and Mabel Hubbard were married in 1877, and although his invention did not help his wife to hear any better, it gained him the Alessandro Volta prize out of which he founded the Volta Bureau in 1887 "for the increase and diffusion of knowledge relating to the deaf."

Bell favored the oral method and the nonsegregation of deaf children so that they could be brought up in normal hearing surroundings.

In 1880 in Milan, under the presidency of the Abbe Tara, a confirmed oralist, the First International Congress of the Teachers of the Deaf recommended, among other things, "That the Pure Oral Method ought to be preferred," and that "no teacher can effectively teach a class of more than ten children in the Pure Oral Method."

The Age of Auditory Training

At the end of the nineteenth century, Dr. Urbantschitsch, a Viennese otologist, attracted much attention by his insistence on the importance of finding out how much residual hearing any deaf child possessed and of exercising such residual hearing to make the deaf child aware of sounds and aware of his own voice. Dr. Kerr Love, the Glasgow otologist, also emphasized the importance of auditory training.

Urbantschitsch attracted the attention of an American otologist, Dr. Goldstein of St. Louis, who was so impressed by this concept that he introduced it to the St. Joseph's School for the Deaf in St. Louis, and in 1914 he founded the Central Institute for the Deaf, an institute which has been and still is a model of co-operation between doctors, teachers, scientists and research workers. Dr. Goldstein's insistence on daily acoustic exercises gave such good results both in hearing and speech that his example was followed throughout the world. In those days, electrical amplifiers were not very effective so he had to rely on speaking tubes, but out of this modest beginning grew the principle of auditory training, and, as we shall see from the next age, there grew with the improvement in hearing tests the idea of finding out what, if any, hearing there was, and, with the help of electrical amplification, making the fullest use of this residual hearing both to get language into and speech out of the deaf child.

The Age of Hearing Tests and Hearing Aids

We must at once acknowledge the debt the deaf world owes to Sir Alexander and the late Lady Irene Ewing for their insistence upon the importance of ascertaining the existence of any hearing in children born deaf. When they started their great work in Manchester before the First World War, there were no such things as audiometers or effective electrical amplifiers. They carried out their tests with rattles, drums, bells, whistles, and pitch pipes; and very effective they were too. The advent of the pure tone audiometer and valve-amplified hearing aids, both of which were perfected after the Second World War, however, made the investigation and exploitation of any residual hearing a much more practical proposition.

At this stage I would like to mention the Peep Show Audiometer, first described by my colleagues Dix and Hallpike in 1947. This form of play audiometry furnishes within half an hour at the most a pure-tone audiogram of all children of average intelligence from the age of 2¹/₂ years. This is an accurate and most effective way of measuring a young child's hearing for pure tones.

With this technique, and with modern transistor hearing aids, it is possible to estimate a child's hearing loss in terms of pure tones, to predict the value of a hearing aid, and to solve some of the tricky problems of high tone deafness which at one time were labeled, for want of a better phrase, "congenital auditory imperception."

The Age of Parental Co-operation

Here again we must mention the pioneer work of the Ewings, who continually stressed the importance of the parents in the early auditory training of the deaf child.

This idea was followed up in a grand way by the John Tracy Clinic of Los Angeles, which specialized in training the parent and the preschool deaf child. I have seen this clinic at work, and many of my patients' parents have enjoyed their correspondence course. But human nature being what it is, not all have profited by the valuable information offered in the course.

Mention must also be made of the remarkable center at Groningen, Holland, under the direction of my friend the physicist H. C. Huizing, who has laid special emphasis on the importance of training any residual hearing that a born-deaf child possesses. At this stage it may be said that the number of children born without any residual hearing is very small indeed.

It is interesting to note that the city of Groningen has been associated with deafness in children for many centuries.

The Age of Early Recognition of Deafness

Again thanks to the Ewings, the idea of a screening test for deaf babies was put forward and through the public health authorities, particularly in Leicester, a screening test carried out by health visitors for babies was established. It was found, for instance, that by the age of six months a child of normal hearing would respond by turning its head sharply in the direction of the sound in response to sounds of such significance to an infant as the rustle of tissue paper and the sound of a spoon in a cup.

Out of this grew the concept that such a test should be automatically administered to any child at risk: that is to say, any child with a history of deafness in the family, any child of a mother who had a febrile illness in the early months of pregnancy (for instance, rubella) and any child who was jaundiced at birth or who had a difficult birth.

Any child who failed to respond to the screening test as described was, after an otological examination to insure that the outer and middle ears were intact, fitted with a hearing aid. I have a vivid recollection of seeing in the Toronto Sick Children's Hospital a child aged eight months under the care of the late Dr. Staunton Wishart with a hearing aid pinned, if you please, to her napkin, and who, as I proved to my own satisfaction, responded happily to sound.

This simple example serves to underline the importance of fitting a hearing aid to an infant as soon as its deafness has been detected. In this way the infant is able to hear what is said to it or to hear its own voice at the time when speech naturally develops. When fitting a hearing aid to an infant or young child, it is important to warn the parents against the possible danger from overstimulation by loud noise. Parents will be well advised to turn the aid down when the child is in a noisy situation.

The Age of Intelligence

I am only human, after all, so I have left the most difficult task almost to the end.

The estimation of the intellectual potential of any child has presented problems from the start in the early years of this century. With the deaf child, tests of intellectual capacity have to be limited to nonverbal or performance tests. Pinter and Paterson in 1917 were the first to publish a special intelligence test for deaf children based on the Binet test, while M. S. Hiskey in 1941 published the Nebraska Test of Learning Aptitude, suitable for deaf children between the ages of 4 and 10 years.

Most of those whose work brings them into regular contact with children born deaf are able, by means that cannot always be put into words, to tell which deaf children are bright and which are dull. And I would like at this point to stress the fact that children born deaf are, apart from their defect, bright, average or dull, as are children with normal hearing.

After receiving a period of special instruction from a skilled teacher of deaf children, all deaf pupils should have the benefit of a special test of intelligence by an educational psychologist. Many of those children who achieve a poor score in their test will be found to have difficulty in learning to lip read, and I am sure that the right thing to do for their future happiness is to cut one's losses and allow them to communicate by signs.

The bright deaf child will take to lip reading like a duck to water and many will be able to take their place in a school for normal hearing children.

For those who are not so bright, much more special training and help is needed, for they will never be able to compete on equal terms with hearing children. They must be allowed to communicate by any means within their intellectual capacity, and they must not be denied the opportunity of signing if they are unable to communicate their thoughts and ideas in any other way.

Without in any way wishing to detract from the importance of the organs of hearing and speech, and the process of receiving and translating language, we must never forget that these organs, necessary though they are for the reception and transmission of speech, are really nothing more than receivers or transmitters. They do not analyse what is heard, nor do they decide what is to be spoken. This is done in the higher centers in the brain and it is to the quality of each individual brain that we should also give some consideration. Although we know quite a lot about the centers for interpreting speech in the temporal lobes of the brain and the center for motor speech in the area described by the French anatomist Broca, too little is known about the quality of the association areas and other reception areas for the special understanding of speech and language.

A great deal has been and is being done in the estimation of the intelligence of children, and I believe that children denied the gift of hearing are as varied in their degree of intelligence as any group of children. A bright deaf child will triumph over his disability in an amazing way, while another child equally deaf will, because of lower intelligence, be unable even with expert help to make much progress in overcoming his defect. We all know the bright deaf child of bright and co-operative parents who suffers but little handicap from his defect. I always remember the child of a surgeon who was born very deaf as the result of maternal rubella. I first saw the little girl when she was eighteen months old. Her mother, a trained teacher, went with the child to Manchester where she spent a year with the Ewings. Then she returned to London, found a small group of other deaf children whom she trained together with her own child. This girl went to an ordinary school and in the end became the head girl. She wanted to follow in her father's footsteps and was eventually admitted to a dental school where she trained and qualified as a dentist by the age of twenty-two. She had but a tiny islet of hearing in the lowest tones, and though she never learned to speak very well she was able to practice successfully as a dentist.

The Otologist and the Deaf Child

Defective hearing may include any hearing loss, from whatever cause, between slight deafness, severe deafness, subtotal deafness and total deafness; the deafness may be congenital or acquired and if severe enough (for instance, subtotal) will, if it is congenital, impair or prevent the acquisition of speech or language.

Before the introduction of the antibiotics and sulphonamides, bilateral otitis media in early childhood, resulting from scarlet fever or measles often caused severe deafness that interfered with the proper development of speech. This is now almost a thing of the past in civilized countries, but still with us is the total deafness which may follow meningococcal meningitis, though if this happens after the natural acquisition of language the effects are not so serious in terms of ability to speak. Children so afflicted form about 10 percent of the population of schools for the deaf, and it is probable that before the days of antibiotics and sulphonamides the proportion was even higher.

A small number of children are deaf because of defects in the sound-conducting part of the auditory apparatus. There is an imperfectly formed outer or middle ear, though the inner ear containing the organ of hearing is intact and functions normally.

The number of such cases must be small, for Ombredanne of Paris, who has collected them for many years, only has about a hundred; and Gavin Livingstone of Oxford who has specialized in the surgical correction of such cases has collected about thirty in the past fifteen years. They must nevertheless be recognized and, of course, dealt with surgically in order to get sound to the normal organ of hearing.

Otosclerosis is a form of conductive deafness that can usually be corrected by surgery; many start before the age of ten and more commonly in the 'teens. Again, this needs to be recognized so that appropriate surgical treatment may be instituted.

Silent effusion into the middle ear may be a cause of deafness, particularly in the young child, which may sometimes be overlooked.

The four causes of childhood deafness that I have just described are located in the sound-conducting part of the auditory mechanism; so there is no doubt that one of the earliest problems to solve when faced with a child with defective hearing is that of deciding which part of the auditory mechanism is affected. If the sound-conducting mechanism is at fault, it can usually be corrected, but if the sound-perceiving part of the auditory mechanism is at fault (that is to say, the end-organ of hearing) then nothing surgically can be done to improve the hearing.

Then there is the group, rapidly dwindling as our ability to test the hearing of young children increases, in whom there appears to be defective appreciation of sound and of the ability to speak without any detectable defect in the sound-conducting or sound-perceiving part of the auditory mechanism. Such cases were sometimes labeled "congenital auditory imperception," but many have now been shown to be a result either of an undetected fault in the organ of hearing (such as high-tone deafness) or of language changes in earliest childhood. There is also a curious but small group wherein twins develop a language of their own. I well remember as a boy the twin sons of a medical friend of my family who would not talk properly and caused the parents much worry until one day their mother, unbeknown to them, entered the nursery and heard one say to the other, "I say, Mother will be cross with us". Only two weeks ago I was consulted by the mother of twin six-year-old girls, whose speech was defective. Their hearing was normal and the speech defect was of the jargon type often seen in twins.

Another small group that Dr. Richard Hunter and I have described under the heading of "sympathetic deafness" may be included in this group, and perhaps I may be allowed to give two illustrations. One was a girl of fourteen on whose father I had operated successfully for otosclerosis. She was an only child, obviously devoted to her father, and she accompanied him every time he came to see me. As his hearing got better, her hearing got worse, and I was asked to examine her. Her ears appeared normal. She has a voice of normal timbre, and though her hearing showed an eighty-decibel loss in each ear for all pure tones she was obviously an accomplished lip reader, even when I spoke to her very softly.

I was naturally rather worried and indeed puzzled about this child, and eventually I agreed to explore her middle ear. This simple procedure revealed no abnormality whatever, but it was at once followed by a complete recovery of hearing in both ears.

One of the other cases deserves mention here; this was the fifteen-year-old son of a lady audiologist. She was divorced and was considering remarriage (as eventually emerged), and the youth was thought to be deaf. Again, he appeared to have profound perceptive deafness—with, however, a normal voice and a remarkable ability to lip-read. The striking resemblance to the first case led me to ask my psychiatric colleague at the National Hospital for Nervous Diseases, Queen Square, Dr. Richard Hunter, to see this boy, and he was able to elicit the rest of the story; the apparent loss of hearing was soon restored. Similar cases have been seen. All were concerned with domestic difficulties and all were readily solved once recognized, though I cannot recommend the exploratory operation in the first case. The only merit in this was that it taught me to recognize and to name "sympathetic deafness".

And now, as I come to the end of my tale, I should like to mention the names of two doctors who took a special interest in deaf-mutism. One was Prosper Ménière who was medical superintendent of a school for the deaf and dumb in Paris.

His claim to immortal fame, however, did not rest on this appointment. He was greatly interested in diseases of the ear and he felt that the inner ear might be responsible for violent attacks of giddiness and sickness associated with deafness and ringing, usually in one ear only. In 1861 he published his belief, on the strength of one individual who had died after exhibiting these symptoms and whose temporal bone and ear he was able to examine. Ever since then this disorder has been known as Ménière's Syndrome or, more recently as Ménière's Disease.

The other doctor who deserves mention is the Irish otologist and oculist, Sir William Wilde. He was a very versatile man and he established an eye and ear infirmary in Dublin in 1843. But his Knighthood was awarded, not for his services to otology, but for his remarkable study of the Irish population in the Irish census. This included a survey of deaf-mutism and a history of its occurrence, not only in Ireland but throughout the world, which he published in an appendix to his text book, *Diseases of the Ear,* published in 1853. One remark in this deserves repetition and is a fitting end to this discourse; I quote;

To me it has always appeared that the patient instructor of the deaf and dumb deserved a reward which nothing earthly could bestow. And the energy, perseverance, philanthropy of those good men and women who have from time to time undertaken in different countries that herculean task of teaching the eye to hear and the hand to speak have only been equalled by the eloquence of those who have advocated the claims which the deaf mute has upon all to whom the Creator has afforded the blessings of speech and hearing.

I wish to acknowledge with gratitude the help given me by Dr. Gorman, librarian of the Royal National Institute for the Deaf, London, whose advice on the history of deafness in children was invaluable.

References

Ballantyne, J. Chalmers. *Deafness.* London: J. & A. Churchill, 1960.

Bender, Ruth. *The Conquest of Deafness.* Cleveland: The Press of Western Reserve University, 1961.

Brain, Lord. *Speech Disorders.* 2nd ed. London: Butterworths, 1965.

Critchley, Macdonald. *The Language of Gesture.* London: Edward Arnold, 1939.

Ewing, I. R. and A. W. G. *Speech and the Deaf Child.* Manchester University Press, 1954.

Ewing, Sir Alexander (ed.). *Educational Guidance and the Deaf Child.* Manchester University Press, 1957.

Whetnall, E. and D.B. Fry. *The Deaf Child.* London: Heinemann, 1964.

Proceedings of the International Course in Paedo-Audiology. University of Groningen, 1953.

Scottish Education Department Command, 7866. *Pupils who are Defective in Hearing.* Edinburgh: Her Majesty's Stationery Office, 1950.

Proceedings of a conference held in Toronto, Canada, October 1964.

"The Young Deaf Child, Identification and Management."
Supplement 206. Acta-Otolaryngologica. Stockholm.

PART II

DIAGNOSIS

TESTING HEARING IN INFANCY AND EARLY CHILDHOOD

THE practicing audiologist takes upon himself a commitment to extend his inquiry into the field of deafness well beyond routine clinical determinations of degrees of deafness and the customary management of habilitation. The audiologist's inquiry starts with the very beginnings of deafness—at birth—and proceeds to continued identification of hearing status following birth. Once the identification of hearing loss is made, the audiologist is confronted furthermore with a commitment that grows out of early identification. He must formulate criteria that will allow him to predict at infancy whether a child's best interests in language development will be served by providing a primary auditory input, a primary visual input, or a combination of both. These three lines of inquiry—detection of suspected hearing loss at birth, follow-up identification of hearing status, and prediction of the best direction habilitation might take—are of deep concern to many audiologists today. The directions these inquiries are taking, or might take, are well worth examining.

Detection of Hearing Loss at Birth

The development of tests of hearing at birth has followed two lines: one is represented by the meticulous kinds of clinical observations being made by Eisenberg *et al.* (1964) and by Murphy (1962), by means of which subtle behavioral responses to various kinds of sounds are noted in a structured environment. The other line consists of more gross screening procedures applicable to large numbers of infants in nonstructured environments. The latter type of test has been reported by Wedenberg (1963), Parr (1962), and Downs and Sterritt (1964), all of whom chose high-frequency signals centering around 3,000 and 4,000 cps, to differentiate hearing disorders from the normal.

The feasibility of this latter kind of gross screening is being demonstrated in the Denver area, where the entire newborn population in eight hospital nurseries is being screened. Approximately 10,000 newborn infants have already been tested in this program. Five infants have definitely been identified and confirmed as being deaf, and the status of others is in the process of verification. The procedure by which the confirmation is made includes repeated observations of behavioral responses and EEG audiometric tests. The heaviest weighting has been given to EEG auditory testing with summing computer techniques, through which confirmation of hearing loss has been obtained by the time the infants reached the age of three months. Three of the infants confirmed deaf were fitted with hearing aids before the age of six months. Their hearing problems were caused respectively by neonatal anoxia, congenital renal disease, and one unknown etiology. The other two infants were children of congenitally deaf parents and did not participate in the habilitation program because of the wishes of the parents. Other infants have been identified immediately after birth as having impaired hearing, but they are not included in the statistics because they were not born in the screening hospitals. These were high-risk cases of rubella, Rh incompatibility, or congenital familial history who were referred to the program. It is thus difficult to derive exact statistics from these numbers, but certainly the incidence of deafness that is being found is at least one in 2,000.

A fairly high rate of false positives is found in the program: $1^1/_2$ percent of the total population fail to respond to the test signal, and 97 percent of these are ultimately cleared.

It should be noted that among the false positives seen at the University of Colorado Medical Center four were diagnosed as having CNS involvement. In each case, the existence of normal peripheral hearing was confirmed by the time the child was three months of age, either by EEG auditory testing, or by behavioral responses, or by both. The percentage of those with CNS involvements who have normal peripheral hearing but who failed to respond at birth does not seem high enough to warrant any conclusion at this time.

The method of screening used in this program was developed at the University of Colorado School of Medicine (Downs and Sterritt, 1964). It utilizes an acoustic signal centered around 3,000 cps at 90 dB (SPL) output. Two instruments have been developed to produce such a signal.[1] The specificity of the signal makes it possible to differentiate from normal hearing those losses that are greater in the high frequencies than in the lows.

The responses of the normal-hearing infant to a signal such as the 3,000 cps noise can easily be observed. They have been variously catalogued as follows (Downs and Sterritt, 1964; Parr, 1962; Wedenberg, 1963): (1) Eye blink, or auro-palpebral reflex. (2) Startle response, resembling the Moro's reflex. (3) Arousal responses (eye-opening, limb movement, stirring). (4) Head turn. (5) Sucking activity. (6) Cessation of movement or vocalization. In the testing program, these responses[2] are carefully classified by the observers, who rate them independently on a five-point scale of intensity:

No Hearing Zone   (1 = No response
                       (2 = Questionable response

Hearing zone   (3 = Slight but definite
                       (4 = Strong
                       (5 = Paroxysmal (Moro's or startle response)

The classification of these responses can be made by well trained, intelligent volunteers, so the program need not be an expensive one. In Denver, sixty members of the Junior League have gone through an intensive training program and are testing in the newborn nurseries of eight hospitals. The training consists of a one-month program during which one or two experienced testers work with one or two novices. A rigid protocol (see Fig. 1) for making observations is followed: the pretesting state of the infant is noted and recorded; then the signal is presented, and each tester independently notes the site of response and the intensity of the response on the five-point scale. Agree-

---

1. The Vicon Apriton (A-Z signal generator), manufactured by the Vicon Instrument Co., 1353 Mesita Road, Colorado Springs, Colorado, and the Rudmose Warblet 3000, manufactured by Tracor, Inc., 6500 Tracor Lane, Austin, Texas.

2. A movie, *Auditory Responses of Newborn Infants,* illustrating these responses is available through Thorne Films, Inc., 1229 University Avenue, Boulder, Colorado (3 minutes, silent, 16 mm., $30.00).

ment between the experienced tester and the novices is necessary; a poor observer who is consistently at variance with the standard observations is quickly weeded out.

NAME (LAST, FIRST)	
PROJECT CASE NO.	
HOSPITAL CASE NO.	HOSPITAL
BIRTHDATE	HOUR BORN
SEX	CRIB/INCUBATOR
FEED TIME (last) (next)	EAR
CLEAR/SUSPECT	RATER

RESPONSE INTENSITY : I, NONE – 2, OBSCURED – 3, WEAK, BUT CLEAR – 4, STRONG – 5, PAROXYSMAL

TEST		CO-RATER	STIMULUS			INFANT	STATE			RESPONSE	
DATE	TIME	INDEP	NAME	REP	DUR	DB	BODY — FACE	EYELIDS	TIME	TYPE	INT
							WHOLE / LIMBS / QUIET / CRY / FRET / VOCAL / GRIM / SUCK / QUIET	OPEN / DROOP / CLOSED		MOVE / SUCK / TURN / LIMB / CESS / WIDEN / LID	

Figure 1. Infant auditory screening test

In order to determine the feasibility of using lay volunteers in a newborn screening program, an analysis of the interobserver reliability of the volunteers was made. A random sample of 154 of the 1,800 most recent newborn test protocols was analyzed. The sample consisted of independent observations made by two or more of the observers. As in our original pilot study by three professional workers, the observations were paired on the basis of the five-point rating scale, resulting this time in 527 pairings of observations. (Most of the infants are given three to six signal presentations at fifteen-second intervals, to derive information on adaptation.) The results are compared in Table I with the original pilot study results. The statistic in the last line was manipulated because it was found that eight infants in the random sample had been tested by training groups of three or four individuals, some of whom were novices. These eight accounted for an inordinate proportion of disagreements, as could be expected; and in order to visualize only the functioning of the routine testers, the pairings accounted for by these eight test protocols were removed from the last statistic.

TABLE I

DISCREPANT RATINGS IN ALL POSSIBLE COMPARISONS
OF TWO OBSERVERS RATING THE SAME RESPONSE

Raters	N		Amount of discrepancy between scores			
		NONE	1	2	3	Critical
Professionals (Pilot Study)	947	585(62%)	325(34%)	34(3.6%)	3(.4%)	100(10.5%)
Random sample, 1500 volunteer ratings	704	563(80%)	134(17.4%)	7(1%)	0	33(5.4%)
Sample minus Training groups	612	514(84%)	95(15.5%)	3(.005%)	0	24(4%)

These results show that in the routine volunteer observations, 84 percent of the paired observations resulted in perfect agreement; in the original professional study only 62 percent of the paired observations were in perfect agreement. Where critical disagreements were concerned—those that cross the hearing—no-hearing line—the volunteer observers disagreed only 4 percent of the time, as against 10.5 percent in the original professional study.

The conclusion is quite apparent that well trained lay people are able to look at babies and to agree on what they see as well as, or better than, professionals. This is an extremely valuable observation, for the use of professional personnel in a mass screening program such as this would be financially prohibitive, considering the low yield involved. The use of volunteers allows the program to be conducted economically in relation to the yield.

It is hoped that further effort will be made to improve and expand the kind of program described, now that its feasibility has been demonstrated.

Testing Procedures for Older Infants

Once means have been found to detect possible hearing loss at birth, it becomes all the more urgent that accurate testing be provided following birth. The most promising technique, and the one that has been most relied upon in our program, is the use of evoked responses. When one considers that the "positives" found in the newborn testing program number $1^1/_2$ percent of the population screened, however, it is evident that such a large number cannot economically be tested with EEG techniques, particularly when 97 percent of the positives are found to have normal hearing. More rapid techniques are required that can be applied, not only by audiologists, but by nurses and doctors in offices and well-baby clinics.

One answer to the need for further screening and follow-up procedures has been provided by the excellent Johns Hopkins film[3] which describes the use of various noisemakers to produce orientation responses in the older infants. Another line of investigation seeks to utilize the measurable acoustic signals that are used in the newborn testing and to obtain norms for infants' responses to these signals. It is the direction of this latter project that will be discussed.

The study currently under way at the University of Colorado Medical Center envisions the development of what might be termed a Baby Auditory Behavior Index (or BABI, if we may be forgiven the acronym), which will describe indices of children's auditory development in relation to acoustic signals of given output and frequency.

Before such a BABI could be described, however, several questions presented themselves: (1) Is the 3000 cps–peaked signal as productive of responses as any other frequency-centered signal? (2) Are there other kinds of measured stimuli that might be used, either independently or as corroboration for a frequency-centered signal? (3) How should signal presentations be given—at random or in a prescribed sequence? To answer these questions a clinical study was designed, using infants from well-baby clinics who are 6 weeks to 24 months old.

The procedure of the study is to have the infant on his mother's lap in a sound room and engage him in quiet play. Two loudspeakers, at 90-degree and 270-degree angles from the infant, are the source of signals. First the infant's name is called through one of the loudspeakers, starting at zero level (re: normal thresh-

---

3. Maryland State Department of Health. 1961. *Auditory Screening for Infants* (film). Baltimore: Division of Maternal and Child Health, 301 West Preston Street.

old), and ascending in five-decibel steps. The first point of true orientation to the speech signal is noted. A bona fide searching movement of the head is the criterion response. Then an ascending warbled puretone signal is given through the loudspeaker, in a sequence of four frequencies—500, 1,000, 2,000, and 3,000 cps—in random order. Orientation points are noted. After that the speech signal is repeated.

Preliminary data from a small population sample of 50 babies indicate that some interesting trends are appearing and are worthy of reporting at this time:

1. The first presentation of any warbled puretone is the critical one for obtaining a response to the lowest possible hearing level. Mean response levels to the frequency series presented at random are:

1st presentation	39 dB
2nd presentation	48 dB
3rd presentation	58 dB
4th presentation	58 dB

These results are logical, considering the expected extinction factor. The results point strongly to the importance of arranging the testing situation so that the first signal presentation can be readily observed and noted.

2. There are no real differences between high and low frequencies as attention-getters for young children. The mean response levels to each frequency on its first presentation were:

500 cps	42 dB
1000 cps	41 dB
2000 cps	32 dB
3000 cps	41 dB

No statistical significance can as yet be attached to these figures, but they tend at this point to refute the traditional observation that low frequencies are more effective for testing young children than high ones.

3. The response to the speech signal is the most consistent indicator of good hearing responses. In all age groups, the standard deviations of the responses to the speech signal do not exceed 7.5 decibels. The mean responses to speech, compared with those to the warbled puretones, are shown in Table II.

TABLE II

COMPARISON BETWEEN MEAN RESPONSES TO
SPEECH AND TO PURE TONES

Age Range	Speech Level	Pure Tone
		(1st Presentation)
6 wks–12 wks	52 dB (δ = 7.5 dB)	75 dB (δ = 9 dB)
3 mo–6 mo	28 dB (δ = 1 dB)	47 dB (δ = 2.4 dB)
6 mo–12 mo	12 dB (δ = 7 dB)	40 dB (δ = 11.3 dB)
12 mo–15 mo	6 dB (δ = 5 dB)	35 dB (δ = 19.5 dB)
15 mo–24 mo	5 dB (δ = 3.4 dB)	26 dB (δ = 11 dB)

The trends shown so far strongly indicate that it will be possible to describe indices of normal auditory behavior, based on measurable signals. The high frequencies evolve as adequate attention-getters and can be used to differentiate subjects with normal hearing from those with high frequency loss. Speech signals emerge as the most effective of any for producing responses at fainter levels, but whether these speech measures represent fine enough screening to differentiate high frequency losses is the question that remains to be answered.

Criteria for Prediction of Function

The detection of hearing loss at these early ages imposes on the audiologist a need for the most critical of judgments: How best can these crucial early years be utilized for the optimum language development of the child? At the present time the assignment of infants and children to a specific type of remedial program is an educated guess founded more on bias than on evidence. Audiologists and educators alike share the responsibility for this situation and should collaborate to find its solution.

It is imperative to initiate research programs directed toward developing indices of the child's potential functioning, based on degree of loss, etiology and site of lesion, intellectual potential, and environmental factors. By the time the infant is six months old the prognosis should be available as to whether the child will best be able to assimilate language through a hearing input; primarily through hearing with supplemental visual clues; or primarily through visual input. At the end of six months' observation, the child can then be directed toward an approach with emphasis on acoustic amplification, toward the acoustic plus lip-reading, toward manual or finger-spelling techniques, or to some combination of these. This kind of information must be available, once we start to reach into infancy to find hearing impairment. Otherwise we compromise our commitment to the deaf.

References

Downs, Marion P., and G. Sterritt. 1964. "Identification Audiometry in Neonates: A Preliminary Report." *J. Auditory Research*, 4:69–80.

Eisenberg, Rita B., E. J. Griffin, D. B. Coursin, and M. A. Hunter. 1964. "Auditory Behavior in the Human Neonate: A Preliminary Report." *J. Speech & Hearing Res.*, 7:245–269.

Murphy, Kevin P. 1962. "Development of Hearing in Babies." *Child and Family*, 1:16–20.

Parr, Walter G. 1962. "Ascertainment of Deafness in Infancy." *Proceedings of the Eighth Conference of Teachers of the Deaf in Australia.* Australian Association of Teachers of the Deaf.

Wedenberg, Erik. 1963. "Auditory Tests on Newborn Infants." *Acta Otolaryng. Suppl.*, 175:1–32.

CHAPTER **3** HARRIET B. MANTELL

PEDIATRIC EVALUATION OF THE DEAF CHILD

THERE are three broad areas in which the pediatrician has a responsibility to the deaf child. The child cannot be diagnosed or treated skillfully unless the pediatrician at least suspects a problem and guides the child and parents in the right direction. The earlier the diagnosis is made and treatment begun, the better chance the child has for rehabilitation. Not every child who fails to respond to sound is deaf. Speaking as a pediatrician in the approach to the differential diagnosis, the possibility of another reason the child does not respond normally to sound must always be considered. The pediatrician is interested medically and psychologically in the whole child attached to the deaf ears. He is concerned with the family upon whose attitudes the child's well-being depends. For the sake of his patient, the pediatrician must be aware of the resources the community has to offer the child.

How do we suspect deafness early in a child's life? The pediatrician has two basic methods: the careful history and observant physical examination. Most deafness can be ascribed to some known cause. Awareness of the historical events that cause or predispose to hearing problems increases the likelihood of finding them. Let us concern ourselves briefly with some of the major ones. First, consider the value of the family history. Since the genetics of deafness will be discussed in several papers that follow in this symposium, it should suffice to say that the pediatrician is alerted by a family history of deafness, thyroid or kidney problems, and such things as white forelocks not produced by the hairdresser's art. Next, information about the prenatal history may be of value. What happened to the mother while she was carrying the baby? Did she have any such infection as German measles or syphilis? Was she given any drugs such as quinine or streptomycin? Were there any complications of pregnancy such as bleeding or toxemia? Was the birth process of the infant normal? Was he premature or of low birth weight? Did he suffer distress during his birth due to prolonged or precipitate labor, injury, or anoxia? In the neonatal period we are interested in whether the child was severely jaundiced and whether he required an exchange transfusion. One of the things that mothers often do not know is that in some hospitals it was routine to give penicillin and streptomycin to every infant who had an exchange transfusion or when the membranes were ruptured more than twenty-four hours before the birth of the baby. It must be recognized that the streptomycin might be an additional factor in these situations. The mother is usually well aware of whether the infant had any respiratory difficulty or required oxygen. Sometimes she possesses more information than appears on the hospital chart. It is important to inquire about infections, since the most frequent cause of conductive impairment in children is inadequately treated otitis media. History should be obtained concerning childhood infections such as mumps and such central nervous system infections as meningitis and encephalitis which can damage the ear. Traumatic injury to the head or ear may be self-explanatory. All of these historical facts are parts of a routine pediatric history if it is acquired carefully, and with an awareness of the causes of deafness the physician should in the majority of cases be alerted to the potential risk of deafness in a specific case. Another point of extreme importance in history-taking is to ask whether the mother thinks the child hears and to take seriously the mother's suspicion that the child cannot hear well. As an example, we had a case in our Multiple Handicap Clinic of a two-year-old boy who was found to be profoundly deaf and of quite normal intelligence on nonverbal psychological tests. On the hospital chart, physicians in the Medical Clinic had noted on at least two occasions during the infancy of this child that the mother had asked that the baby's hearing be tested because she thought he could not hear. To our extreme chagrin, it was also recorded that the examiners thought the child could hear. Little did they know that it was this baby's acute visual alertness they had tested. It was virtually impossible to sneak a tuning fork or anything else along side this bright-eyed boy without his reacting. It is still a mystery what in particular made this mother, who had two older normal children, suspect her infant's hearing defect.

We do know there are a number of questions that can be asked that cause us to respect and learn from the mother's observations. Was this a newborn who did not startle at a loud noise, who slept through all kinds of commotion? Did he not stop crying when she spoke to him or did he fail at six months to turn to the sound of his mother entering the room but act surprised when she appeared in view? When this mother expressed concern that her child did not respond to what she said and did not begin to say words, she was told that he was mentally retarded. Had the examining physician observed the baby's behavior more closely and listened to the mother, he would have been able to spare the family the grief of misdiagnosis of mental retardation and to start the appropriate treatment for a deaf child. The value of the pediatric history depends upon the questioner's patience and understanding of the factors that should alert one to the possibility of problems. While remembering that most children with compromising histories turn out to be normal, it is also important to note that the converse is sometimes true. Sometimes deafness appears without any prior warning, and the cause cannot be picked up by history.

Attention must then be turned in these cases to the physical examination for further hints. Certain more obvious defects noted on physical examination are associated with hearing deficit. Every child observed to have cerebral palsy, cleft palate, or speech defects is entitled to a careful hearing assessment. This also is true for children who appear mentally slow because it is easy to confuse hearing defects and mental retardation and because in some children the same brain insult is responsible for both an intellectual and a hearing deficit. If the examination reveals multiple congenital anomalies that are visible, one might entertain the suspicion that the child might have congenital deafness as well, particularly if the external ear is malformed. In light of the ever-present possibility that a mother may have had rubella unknown to herself, which could affect her unborn child, we need to be suspicious of hearing loss when we find other symptoms of the rubella syndrome, such as microcephaly, congenital heart disease and eye problems. The hypothyroid child who is recognized by his lethargy, dry skin, constipation, umbilical hernia, poor development and laboratory tests is another candidate for hearing assessment as a routine part of his care. But for the child who has nothing else wrong with him and has given us no clues in the past history, we have to rely on our knowledge of normal growth and development of children in order to spot the developmental deviations that indicate hearing loss.

To Arnold Gesell, we owe an important and useful concept that the development of an infant proceeds along clearly defined and predictable lines, so that marked deviations from these are usually significant. A British pediatrician, Dr. R. S. Illingsworth, has applied the work of Gesell and others to everyday pediatric practice, adding some pithy observations and judgments from his long experience of examining normal and abnormal children. I use and highly recommend Illingsworth's book, *The Development of the Infant and Young Child,* in which he describes minute details at week-by-week intervals of what can be observed in the infant during a pediatric examination. There are many excellent photographs of babies in characteristic attitudes that illustrate steps in development and responses to stimuli. Included in the features of development are the responses to sound and voice and the vocalizations to be expected of the infant. To Dr. Ruth Griffith, an English psychologist, we are indebted for a Developmental Scale that is very useful for young babies. Taking an example from our clinic, Figure 1 illustrates a Griffith's Developmental Scale profile on a 6-month-old baby with rubella syndrome. Note that the Griffith's Scale is divided into five areas—Locomotor, Personal-Social, Hearing and Speech, Eye-Hand, and Performance—and that a developmental quotient can be expressed for each of these. This is figured in the same way as the intelligence quotient—i.e., 100 indicates an average performance for the age of the child. As is clearly noted, this child is severely retarded. Observe that while he is far below his age level in all areas, he is lowest in the hearing and speech areas and we are pretty sure he is deaf. For comparison, Figure 2 is an example from Ruth Griffith's book, *The Abilities of Babies,* showing the typical profile of a "normal" deaf child. You will note the deep trough in the hearing and speech area and a lesser drop in the personal-social scale which is thought to be due to the failure to hear and comprehend the spoken instructions and urging of the mother

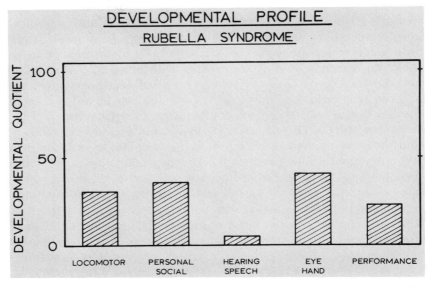

Figure 1. Development scale profile of a six-month-old infant with rubella syndrome, showing severe retardation in all categories.

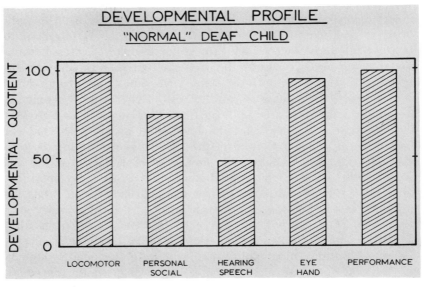

Figure 2. Developmental scale profile of typical "normal" deaf child. Hearing and speech areas and personal social scales are primarily affected.

while the locomotor, eye-hand, and performance areas are unaffected.

We have so far discussed our efforts to discover a deaf child by history and by physical examination. Occasionally we find another puzzling problem in a child who may not be deaf at all in actuality but who is not responding to sound in a normal fashion. This is particularly true with the youngest children, and the differential diagnosis may not be simple. For reasons of their own, many children decide that they are not a bit interested in co-operating with the testing situation. Also, there are children who subsequently turn out to be perfectly normal who at some stage are not at the level one expects for their age, possibly because of some recent illness or just their own individual pattern of spurts and plateaus in development that leaves them at a different spot from most children their age. Some of the most puzzling children to figure out and to treat are those with central nervous system abnormalities. Even with neurological consultation, psychological testing by someone experienced in detecting perceptual problems, and the advice of an educator sophisticated in regard to learning disabilities, one is often left with only a tentative diagnosis. Observation of the child's response to his medical and educational treatment then becomes an integral part of the ongoing diagnosis. Mental retardation is a condition commonly confused with deafness. The inattention and lack of responsiveness of the retarded child often seems to be inability to hear. One thing we found was that it may take a retarded child a long time to respond to any stimulus, and that if one waits long enough without muddying the waters by introducing something new, the retarded child may respond. A psychotic or autistic child may first come to our attention because of lack of response to sound or to speech. The seriousness of this makes it imperative to get psychiatric consultation. It is well to be aware of some of the outstanding features of these children, such as their preference of things to people, their use of people as if they were inanimate objects or tools, preoccupation with spinning objects and, if it is present, a small area of normal or even superior ability accompanying a generalized lack of performance.

The last item in the differential diagnosis brings us to psychosocial deprivation. In the past, much was made of the unstimulated institutionalized baby. Lately we have come to realize that there are homes in which parents are so lacking themselves in intelligence, education, or sensitivity, or are so pressured by life, that they don't give their children the stimulation essential to normal child development. These children also do not know how to respond normally to speech and sound. I have so far discussed what the pediatrician can do in regard to the diagnosis of the deaf child. I hope it is quite clear that I do not think the pediatrician should do this alone and unaided. I count myself fortunate that I work as part of a clinical team that includes a speech pathologist, psychologist, social worker, public health nurse, and educator and have available consultations in all of the departments of our hospital.

As an example, we recently saw a 6½-year-old girl. The history revealed that the mother suffered severe high blood pressure during pregnancy, and at birth the baby was small for the length of gestation and smaller than her two older sisters were at birth. During her early infancy she was irritable, cried a lot for no obvious reason, and her development in all areas was slow. All her life she has had frequent colds, some with ear infections, and she habitually breathes through her mouth. Her speech was difficult to understand and she tended to talk too loud. She was a shy, fearful, immature girl who was spending a second year in kindergarten but still had trouble keeping up with the other children and was unable to concentrate very long on any one thing.

On physical examination, she was in the lower percentiles for height and weight, and her tympanic membranes were lacking a normal light reflex but were not injected. The speech pathologist reported that her audiogram showed about a 40-decibel bilateral conductive hearing loss. Her articulation was typical of a child with a hearing deficit, and there was a marked language delay. The psychologist found that on the Stanford-Binet, which penalizes lack of verbal skills, she tested in the retarded range, but on the performance items of other tests she showed evidence of more ability. Our nurse found her vision to be 20/50 in both eyes, using an eye chart, and she was given an appointment for a complete eye examination.

Socioeconomically, the family was of quite a low level educationally and financially, though sincerely interested in the child's welfare. Our ENT consultant advised adenoidectomy and decongestants. Now what will happen next? We will have to retest her hearing after surgery to see whether it has improved sufficiently or whether she needs further medical or surgical treatment, possibly a hearing aid. Glasses may quite possibly be prescribed to help her vision. We have recommended a formal speech and language program. The family will be guided to help her emotional problems and to provide more enriching experiences. What will be the effect of all this on her ability to learn and her "I.Q." score? Next fall, will she fit best in a class for mentally retarded, a hard-of-hearing program, or neither? After trying all of the known techniques and then retesting the child, we will be in a better position to judge.

This brings us to what I believe is the most important contribution of the pediatrician, that is, to see the deaf child as a deaf child with many needs, all of which are important to how successful a person he turns out to be. He needs the education appropriate to his degree of handicap and someone to remind the community if he has slipped into some crevice between the resources available. He needs opportunities to develop his personality and satisfying relationships with others, and parents who accept and understand him and his handicap. The parents may need support in regard to their feelings about producing a deaf child and their reactions of overprotection or denial that interfere rather than help their child. This fall we saw a child who did not wear his hearing aid and was an impossible behavioral problem in school. At the root of this trouble we felt was the parents' pain and guilt that he was the third of their three children to have some sort of inborn problem. They also happened to be people to whom appearances were very important. Therefore, in many subtle ways they not only did not encourage but actually discouraged their child from using the hearing aid he needed. Little wonder he was a behavioral problem. Every child is entitled to the medical treatment that will help him and to adequate evaluation in every area that has help to offer him. The pediatrician stands as a guide and co-ordinator. In regard to any one child, one may need to consider the views of the parents, the otolaryngologist, the audiologist, the teacher, the speech therapist, the neurologist, the psychologist, the social worker, the scout leader, the camp counsellor—have I left anyone out? Someone needs to be a traffic director with the over-all interests of the child paramount. I offer the pediatrician.

THE OTOLOGIST'S RESPONSIBILITY TOWARD DEAF CHILDREN

THE early history of the development of responsibility for the deaf and hard-of-hearing child is, in very general terms, the history of the development of special education for the deaf. There was, for example, interest in eighteenth-century French scientific circles in what we now describe as "auditory training." The otologists Wilde and Toynbee, the one perhaps better known as the father of Oscar Wilde and the other as the parent of the Toynbee maneuver, each played a part in the development of our understanding of deaf-oral education. In 1911, Kerr Love, quoted by Whetnall and Fry (1964), claimed that the medical profession was neglecting the deaf child, and at the same time he made some very unprophetic statements concerning the relative uselessness of the study of temporal bones taken from the deaf. Max Goldstein, founder of the Central Institute for the Deaf, was another medical authority who stressed the importance of acoustic or auditory training. Much more recently the Ewings of Manchester taught us the feasibility of the early measurement of hearing and the feasibility of detecting hearing defects in the infant; they abruptly shifted our emphasis in the direction of early *detection* and *diagnosis* rather than rehabilitation. Their work was followed in London by that of Dr. Edith Whetnall, who used methods similar to those introduced by the Ewings for this new venture, the early detection and diagnosis of deafness.

It is appropriate at this point to mention briefly some other relatively new developments related to the problems of the deaf or hard-of-hearing child. We shall be hearing more during this symposium about electrodermal and EEG audiometry as well as electronic data processing. These test methods may, for the sake of immediate convenience, be described as "objective" because, as they were introduced, there were high hopes they would prove to be just that—objective tests of hearing requiring little or no co-operation on the part of the test subject. Electrodermal audiometry has not lived up to expectations in terms of its objectivity or its feasibility, but the use of evoked potentials, together with a response averaging system, holds great promise of success and may provide a diagnostic test method approaching true objectivity.

Another subject of consuming interest to all of us interested in the deaf and hard-of-hearing child is that of hearing aids, and it is probably with respect to their use by the deaf child that most recent changes in hearing-aid technology or application have taken place. Almost the only change the deaf adult has seen is that hearing aids have become very much smaller and less efficient. We have learned, however (again thanks in large part to Edith Whetnall), that there is almost no deaf or hard-of-hearing infant too young to use a hearing aid. Four or five years used to be considered the age at which a hard-of-hearing child could be introduced to the idea of using a hearing aid; but educators have pointed out that a child of four or five has already passed his peak learning period. In recognition of this fact, it is now customary to try to detect deafness and fit hearing aids as early as possible during the first year or eighteen months of life; in this way, speech and language development often progress rapidly and ground is gained which might otherwise be lost irretrievably if the hearing aid were to be withheld for several years.

Until just a few years ago it was customary to fit deaf children with only one hearing aid; now, almost as frequently, binaural aids are used because of the attendant gains in usefulness resulting probably from improvements in localization of sound and improved speech discrimination under noisy listening conditions. There is fairly general agreement that even the much abused "Y" cord is often better than a monaural hearing system. In somewhat the same vein, there is growing recognition that for the deaf or hard-of-hearing child who shows marked loudness recruitment a hearing aid with automatic gain control will be superior to one lacking this output-control feature.

One of the most exciting new areas of interest where outstanding advances are being made is that of hereditary deafness. Stevenson and Cheeseman (1956) investigated the families of 421 cases of congenital deafness in Northern Ireland. Their original work must be consulted for complete details, but a few of their conclusions are of vital interest to us. Fewer than 1 percent of marriages in the general population are consanguineous; the corresponding figure for this group of 421 cases was 11 percent. 73 percent of their cases were products of unions between normally hearing parents with no family history of deafness; 24 percent were from deaf parents and the remainder resulted from unions in which only one partner had defective hearing. Chung, Robinson, and Morton (1959) later carried out a detailed analysis of the Stevenson-Cheeseman data; in general terms it seemed probable that more than 60 percent of the cases of hereditary deafness were homozygous for autosomal recessive genes while 22 percent were heterozygous for dominant mutant genes. Treacher-Collins's syndrome and Waardenburg's syndrome are familiar clinical examples of dominant genetic types. Other recognized genetic types include retinitis pigmentosa and vestibulocerebella ataxia; another is Pendred's syndrome, which consists of a congenital deafness with goiter developing in middle childhood. Many more genetic types are being and will be worked out.

It is unnecessary to recount the various ways in which surgery is now sometimes able to help some deaf children. Suffice it to say that, often with a diagnostic assist of immeasurable value from the new radiographic technic of multiple tomographic sections, we are now able to recognize and correct surgically more middle-ear anomalies than was previously possible.

Rather than immediately discuss the otologist's responsibilities, I have listed some of those areas where the otologist must display some measure of responsibility and competence if his practice includes deaf children. His responsibilities fall into two areas: diagnosis of deafness (together, of course, with medical or surgical treatment where possible) and parent counseling.

In the matter of the diagnosis of communication problems in infants and children we are no longer satisfied with a simple ear examination and a hearing test; many other types of work-up are gaining acceptance as essential, including general medical, metabolic, neurological, psychological, and now genetic studies. The otologist is clearly not to be expected to carry out all of these examinations himself, but it is equally clear that if he works in this area he must be well trained in his own field (including the physiology and pathology of hearing, the prevention and treatment of deafness), and he must know a good deal about these other subjects such as the normal development of speech and language, audiology, and the rehabilitation of the deaf (particularly concerning the availability of local resources). He does not have to be an audiologist, but he must know a good deal about the utility and feasibility of various types of hearing tests; he cannot be a geneticist but he must be conversant with the advances being made in genetics. Present-day otologists working with deaf children have these skills and they are in a good position to co-ordinate the type of multi-faceted diagnostic evaluation a noncommunicating child requires; and it may well be that inadequate co-ordination contributes significantly to our evident failure to diagnose and rehabilitate sufficiently early.

Whether or not a firm diagnosis can be reached, the parents of a deaf or hard-of-hearing child require counseling very early in the course of their exposure to the often-cold light of a clinical investigation; with reference to this need, a "Report of the Sub-Committee on Family Counseling and Parent Education" (by Herschel L. Allen and Mary L. Thompson, January, 1965) of the Committee on Hearing Impaired of the Welfare Council of Metropolitan Chicago states:

It is almost universal that parents experience great fear and anxiety in first learning that they have a child with a physical, mental or emotional handicapping condition. Therefore, the Committee strongly believe that it is at this time when services to parents of hearing impaired children are vital. By providing adequate early service to these parents, problems which might have developed later can be prevented. Experience has shown that these problems are much more difficult to deal with if they are not attended to early. The counseling services may be provided in a variety of settings and by a variety of professional persons. But parents usually turn to a medical practitioner who probably has been involved in establishing the diagnosis of hearing impairment. There is a definite need for personnel within the medical setting to counsel with parents when they first experience the impact of learning that their child is handicapped.

Logically, this counseling is the responsibility of the otologist who makes the diagnosis or the decision concerning disposition; we are thus given yet another reason why the otologist of today must be conversant, if only to a limited extent, with much of the subject matter I have listed. Parent counseling should not stay with the otologist; but that is where it must start.

Two major areas have been indicated where the otologist has important responsibilities towards the deaf and hard-of-hearing child: First, he plays a major role in the ever-increasing complexities of diagnostic evaluation and in the medical and surgical treatment of hearing problems; secondly, he initiates that urgent but often neglected process of parent counseling. These are responsibilities the otologist already recognizes; but there is another responsibility which he sometimes overlooks and whose importance should be stressed. The process of detection, diagnostic appraisal, treatment, and rehabilitation of the deaf child is growing increasingly complex; it can be carried out only by a team of professionals of which the otologist is a member; but that team of professionals is becoming very concerned that the standards of hearing evaluation and rehabilitation of the deaf be improved. The otologist may be the logical person to co-ordinate the operation of the diagnostic-treatment-counseling team; by the same token, he should assume greater responsibility for co-ordinating efforts to *improve* the diagnostic facilities available to infants and children.

It is a sad commentary on the times we live in as we are counseled against assuming responsibility in this area because co-ordination sometimes is claimed to be unnecessary and the work involved too great. Only as otologists accept responsibility in this direction will we be able to out-date the following words, contained in a report to the Secretary of the Department of Health, Education and Welfare by his Advisory Committee on the Education of the Deaf.

The American people have no reason to be satisfied with their limited success in educating deaf children and preparing them for full participation in our Society. Less than half of the deaf children needing specialized pre-school instruction are receiving it. The average graduate of a public residential school for the deaf—the closest we have to generally available "high schools" for the deaf—has an eighth grade education. Seniors at Gallaudet College, the nation's only college for the deaf, rank close to the bottom in performance on the Graduate Record Examination.

To meet that responsibility, (in the education of the deaf) we must move promptly and vigorously on several fronts. Of prime importance, we must expand and improve our programs of *early attention* to the deaf child.

The infant with a hearing defect or a potential hearing defect should have a better chance of being identified in the early months of life and be put in touch with better and more generally available clinical facilities and multidisciplinary services for diagnosis and evaluation. Parents of deaf children need more readily available counsel, guidance and instruction.

References

Chung, C. S., O. W. Robison, and N. E. Morton. 1959. "A Note on Deaf-Mutism." *Am. J. Human Genet.,* **23**:357–366.

Fisch, L. (Ed.). 1964. *Research in Deafness in Children.* Oxford: Blackwell Scientific Publications.

Kerr Love, J. 1911. *The Deaf Child.* Baltimore: John Wright & Sons.

Stevenson, A. C., and E. A. Cheeseman. 1956. "Hereditary Deaf Mutism with Particular Reference to Northern Ireland." *Ann. Human Genetics,* **20**:177–231.

Whetnall, Edith, and D. B. Fry. 1964. *The Deaf Child.* Springfield, Illinois: C. C Thomas.

CHAPTER **5** ROBERT GOLDSTEIN

ELECTROPHYSIOLOGIC EVALUATION OF HEARING

MANY kinds of electrophysiologic responses have been used as indexes of hearing, but the only two that have achieved popular clinical usage are the electrodermal response and the electroencephalic response. Audiometry based on these two responses developed historically in an interweaving and alternating pattern.

In the early 1900s, suggestions were being offered about the utilization in audiometry of the sensory-evoked skin resistance and potential changes described late in the previous century by Féré and Tarchanoff, respectively. Successful application of electrodermal audiometry was nevertheless reported only in occasional individual cases, and no one reported successful application to the communicatively impaired child.

Shortly after the early work on EEG in this country in the mid-thirties, interest was stirred in utilizing the EEG changes in response to sound for audiometric purposes. Several attempts were made to test young children by means of electroencephalic audiometry. These attempts were frustrated by the tendency of a child to adapt rapidly to auditory stimuli; the child would react only occasionally after an initial response and then only to very intense stimuli. Technical difficulties, particularly electrical interference, also added to the frustration.

Shortly after the Second World War, thanks largely to the

The preparation of this paper was supported in part by research grant NB–04799 and grant 5–K3–NB–25,383 from the National Institute of Neurological Diseases and Blindness of the Public Health Service.

work of the Johns Hopkins group, there was a resurgence of electrodermal audiometry, or EDA, this time with concentration on the testing of children. With the application of conditioning technics, EDA became more effective.

The great need and desire for a successful objective test for young children led to a wave of unrealistic enthusiasm for EDA. Gradually, however, clinicians began to realize that EDA was least effective with the children for whom it was needed most, particularly for the very young, for the unintelligent, and for the unco-operative children. EDA still has its place in the testing of some children and adults, but in most clinics throughout the world EDA is not commonly used in the battery of tests for assessing auditory function in children.

At the same time that EDA was on the wane as a popular clinical test, EEA (electroencephalic audiometry) was regaining popularity, largely through the work of Derbyshire. Most of the previous technical difficulties had been overcome, and improved testing technics did allow the observation of fairly consistent responses to stimuli close to threshold. In addition, the success of EEA did not seem to be limited by the age or intelligence of the child. Lack of co-operation could be controlled by sedation or anesthesia, which do not seem to depress electroencephalic responses as they do electrodermal responses.

Future experiments and clinical experience may again reverse the historical trend. For the moment, however, the greatest concentration of interest and effort is on electroencephalic rather than electrodermal audiometry. Consequently, the remainder of this chapter will be devoted to the use of EEA in the measurement of hearing in communicatively handicapped children.

Electroencephalic audiometry has taken two common forms. In one, changes in the basic electroencephalogram or EEG in response to single acoustic stimuli are used as indicators of hearing. In a more recent form, averaged responses in the EEG to multiple stimuli are used as indicators of hearing.

Basic to both forms of EEA is the recording of ongoing brainwave activity in the form of an EEG. Electrode placements similar to those used for recording EEG for neurologic evaluation can be used for conventional EEA, or electrodes on or near the vertex can be referred to more peripheral ones on the scalp, or on the mastoid or earlobe.

A child can be tested awake but a young child who is awake is

frequently difficult to restrain for long periods. It is often pref-
erable, therefore, to test a child while he is asleep. Sleep in many
instances has to be promoted through sedation, sometimes light
anesthesia.

The nature of the electroencephalic response and responsitivity
is somewhat dependent on the nature of the basic EEG activity,
which in turn depends largely on the state of sleep or wakefulness of the child. An exception to this generality occurs during
Stage I of sleep following a period of deeper sleep, a stage usually
accompanied by rapid eye movements. During this stage of light
sleep, the children are particularly refractory to acoustic stimulation. The basic EEG pattern is very similar during Stage I of
light sleep following an initial period of wakefulness, yet during
this period responses are elicited rather easily.

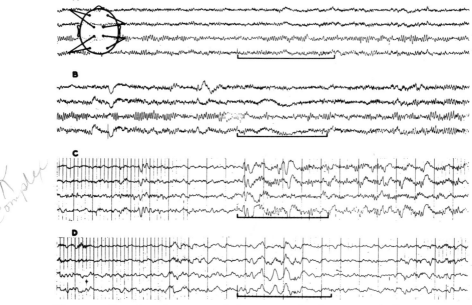

Figure 1. Sample electroencephalogram and electroencephalic responses
from a ten-year-old child. The line under each strip indicates the duration of
the pure-tone stimulus (approximately 5 seconds). A and B early stages of
test, child awake; C and D: child asleep (see text for description of
responses). (From F. B. Withrow, Jr., and Robert Goldstein, in *Laryngoscope,*
68, 1676).

Figure 1 illustrates some of the kinds of changes one might

expect in response to sound. The dark line under each strip shows the duration of the pure tone that was used as the stimulus. In strip A the changes are minimal and the low-frequency or slow wave about halfway through the tone might actually have been an electrodermal reaction from the scalp. In strip B, the response is quite clear. The ongoing 10 per sec or alpha rhythm suddenly disappears within a few tenths of a second after the tone begins. The alpha activity remains suppressed until several seconds after the tone is discontinued.

In strip C, taken while the child was in light sleep a clear response known as the K-complex occurs. It is a series of rather low-frequency or slow waves on which some faster activity is superimposed. The EEG in this particular instance does not return to the original pattern, even with the cessation of the tone.

In strip D, taken while the child was in moderately deep sleep, the response is a series of very low-frequency or slow waves. When the tone is discontinued, the record becomes flattened or suppressed. Then, after about three seconds, the pattern begins to resume its prestimulus form.

Other kinds of responses can also occur, but these are the ones most commonly seen.

If all responses were as dramatic or as obvious as they are in this figure, measurement of hearing by EEA would be very effective in all instances. Responses, however, are seldom this dramatic. Figure 2 illustrates the kinds of responses that one is more likely to observe. In strip A there is only a portion of the K-complex obvious shortly after the onset of the tone. In strip B there is an increase in the ongoing slow-wave activity and in strip C there is a reduction in the ongoing slow-wave activity. Sometimes the responses are even less obvious.

Because of the ordinary clarity of responses, the tester is often hard pressed to make judgments of responses and to determine thresholds. His subjective judgments enter into the test situation. Thus, despite the objective nature of the responses, the test itself can be quite a subjective one. There are ways by which the test can be made more objective by controlling the judgments of the tester. The point to be stressed is that one cannot automatically assume that he is performing objective audiometry when he is doing an EEA, unless he takes great care to maintain the objectivity of his judgments of responses.

When test procedures are objective, threshold measurements derived from EEA correspond to threshold measurements derived

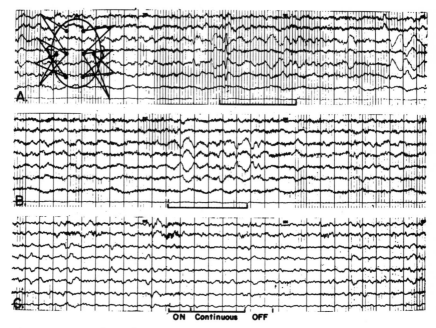

Figure 2. Examples of common electroencephalic responses (see text for description of responses). The line under each strip indicates the duration of the pure-tone stimulus (approximately 5 seconds). In strip C this line was marked off in segments to illustrate the time periods that were considered "on," "continuous" and "off." (From Robert Goldstein, David Kendall, and Bess E. Arick, in *J. Speech and Hearing Disorders*, **28**, 346.

from tests in which voluntary responses are used as indicators of hearing, within the clinical error of each test.

Only one kind of inference can be made from thresholds measured reliably by any technic, and that is about the integrity of the peripheral auditory mechanism. If thresholds measured by EEA are poorer than normal, then all that can be said is that some portion of the peripheral auditory mechanism is not functioning properly: the external ear, the middle ear, the inner ear, or the auditory nerve is faulty, or perhaps several of these components could be affected at the same time. The threshold measures tell nothing about how the brain handles the auditory signal, even though the brain's responses are used to measure the auditory thresholds.

If all kinds of reliable tests yield essentially the same threshold data, then of what particular clinical value is EEA? First of all it is not always possible to determine auditory sensitivity in young children from behavioral responses or from other electrophysiologic indexes, such as electrodermal responses. EEA thresholds can also serve to confirm thresholds that were determined with considerable uncertainty by other procedures.

Knowledge of thresholds provides the clinician with valuable information for making a diagnosis or for guiding a child with a disorder of communication into the appropriate educational channels. But thresholds seldom tell the whole story. Is there anything about the *nature* of the electroencephalic responses that reveals something more about nature of a disorder of communication in an infant or young child? Information along this line is very limited. Nothing in the response patterns, for instance, can indicate whether a very young child is deaf, aphasic, mentally retarded or emotionally disturbed. Nor can the responses tell what part of the brain is affected, even in children with obvious brain damage.

Several years ago, we reported a study on a group of thirty-four children whose organic problems were inferred to be only peripheral, or only central, or a combination of both. These groups and their response characteristics are shown in Table I. The "deaf"

TABLE I

ELECTROENCEPHALIC RESPONSE FEATURES WHICH TEND TO DISTINGUISH AMONG CHILDREN WITH DISORDERS OF COMMUNICATION.

Diagnostic category	Tendency for scores to increase with intensity level	Nature of 'on' responses	Ratio of 'on' to 'continuous' scores
Deaf	Strong	K-complex	Greater than 1 (1.38)
Deaf and Other	No tendency	Almost equal distribution among K, increase in slow, decrease in slow	Slightly less than 1 (0.88)
Other	Moderate tendency	Increase in slow and decrease in slow	Considerably less than 1 (0.69)

group comprises those children who presumably had only a peripheral impairment and were hard of hearing or deaf. The "other" group children had normal auditory sensitivity but were aphasic, mentally retarded, emotionally disturbed, or had some unclassifiable condition, presumably because of some central nervous system lesion. The children in the "deaf and other" group presumably had both peripheral and central lesions.

One of the characteristics that appeared to distinguish the hard-of-hearing or deaf children from the others was the tendency for these children to show increasing responsivity with increasing strength of stimulation. The children with some presumed central nervous system impairment seemed to give almost as many responses to weak stimuli as to strong stimuli. A second distinguishing feature is the nature of the electroencephalic responses that occurred within the first one and one half seconds after the onset of the stimulus. Children with impaired ears but normal brains tended to show the K-complex as a common "on" response, while children with impaired brains but normal ears seldom showed the K-complex; increases or decreases in ongoing slow activity were more common responses in these children. A third distinguishing feature is related to the latency of response. The hard-of-hearing children showed a larger proportion of responses during the first one and one half seconds of the stimulus than they did during the remaining three and one half seconds. In children with presumed central nervous system lesions, the reverse seemed to be true, i.e., it seemed to take a longer time to initiate a response in these children.

Other response features helped to a much lesser extent to distinguish among these children. Even the three features shown in this table, however, have limited diagnostic utility. They do tend to distinguish between *groups* of children but are not as definitive with individual children.

EEA rarely, if ever, provides conclusive diagnostic information by itself. Its results must be correlated with other test results and observations to help in formulating a diagnosis.

Because of its great potential as an auditory test, ways are being sought of improving the utility of EEA. The most significant step in this direction has been the adaptation of the so-called average-response computer for audiometric purposes.

Under most circumstances, the amplitude of evoked responses diminishes rapidly with successive auditory stimuli. The background EEG meanwhile continues at an essentially constant level, and compared with response amplitude, the background EEG voltage is relatively high. As a consequence, during the course of testing it is usually difficult to detect in the EEG a distinct change in the background pattern that might have been induced by auditory stimulation.

With an average-response computer one can store a fixed portion of electroencephalic activity following the onset of each stimulus. Presumably, the background EEG is random in time with respect to the stimulus, and successive additions to the background potentials should, theoretically, add to zero or a straight line graphically. The very small evoked responses which, it is hoped, are consistent in pattern and time-locked to the stimulus should add to each other and eventually accumulate sufficient voltage to be displayed as a characteristic response. The amplitude and form of response will depend on many factors, such as the rate, number, and intensity of stimuli; the state of wakefulness or sleep; or the psychic state of the subject or patient.

An electrode attached to the vertex of the head referred to an electrode on the earlobe or mastoid seems to provide as sensitive a lead as any for detecting the small responses to the repetitive stimulation that is used in computer EEA.

Studies on normal awake adults and older children have yielded a rather characteristic pattern in response to short-duration stimuli and are shown in Figure 3. The responses are believed to correspond to the K-complex noted in the regular EEG tracings. The responses from children are approximately the same as those elicited from adults, except for the possibility of longer latencies and larger amplitudes.

The amplitude of the averaged evoked response does diminish with diminishing strength of the stimulus. In Figure 4, such a diminution of amplitudes with weaker levels of stimulation can be seen. In order to measure threshold, one would look for the weakest stimulus which would just barely elicit an averaged evoked response.

Just as with the electroencephalic response to a single stimulus, the averaged evoked response is not always identifiable.

The form of the response will vary with the state of the child. Sleep in particular makes a distinct change in its form. Figure 5 illustrates this for three children in natural or induced sleep. A Typical adult response is included for comparison. The most prominent feature of the sleep response is a large negative peak just beyond 300 msec.

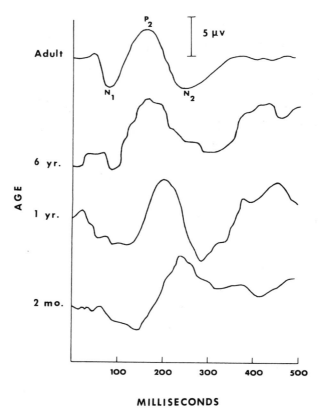

Figure 3. The averaged evoked response from adults and children of various ages. All tracings are responses to stimuli of approximately 50 dB sensation level. Up = vertex positive with respect to earlobe, in this and all following figures. (From Lloyd Price and Robert Goldstein, in J. *Speech and Hearing Disorders*, **31**, 251.

In these illustrations, attention is given to what are usually designated as late components of the averaged evoked responses, i.e., those which occur 50 msec or later after the onset of the stimulus. We have been able to see earlier components, one with a peak latency of 18–20 msec, at threshold hearing levels in normal-hearing adults and older children. Others have also reported early components, but these have been questioned as probably being of myogenic origin. At this time we cannot say whether the vertex-negative potential which we see at about 18–20 msec is neurogenic, myogenic, or a combination of both. Regardless of its

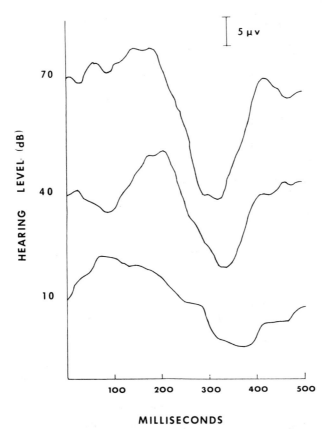

Figure 4. Averaged evoked response showing effects on N₂ (large negative peak at about 300 msec) of intensity of stimuli. All three tracings were from a 2¹/₂-year-old boy medicated with Nembutal. (From Lloyd Price and Robert Goldstein, in *J. Speech and Hearing Disorders*, **31**, 251.)

origin, we believe that this and other early components may soon be shown to have great audiometric utility.

Although EEA with averaged evoked responses is beset by many of the same difficulties one encounters with the earlier form of EEA, it still holds more promise as an effective audiometric tool. Averaged responses to many stimuli are more frequently identified than individual responses to single stimuli, and patterns seem to have more consistency to them so that deviations in them may someday be linked with specific disorders of communication. At that future date, the audiologist may be able to

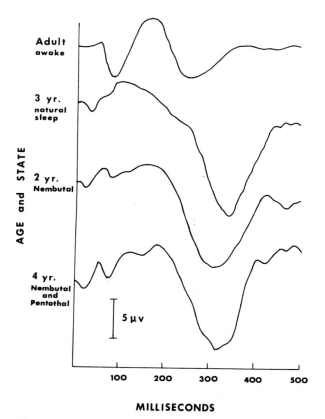

Figure 5. Averaged evoked responses showing effect of sleep, either natural or induced with Nembutal, or with Nembutal and Pentothal. (From Lloyd Price and Robert Goldstein, in *J. Speech and Hearing Disorders*, **31**, 252.)

provide information in addition to threshold measures to help the physician make a more accurate diagnosis and to help the teacher to plan an appropriate educational program for a particular young child.

EEA in any form at the present time, however, can tell us through threshold measures only about the integrity of the total peripheral auditory mechanism. Much research is needed before EEA can tell us about the integrity of the central nervous system and about the potential for development of verbal communication through appropriate educational therapy.

PSYCHOEDUCATIONAL EVALUATION

EVALUATING educational potential of a young deaf child is not an easy task: it is what a child can or cannot do with whatever residual hearing he has that we should like to be able to predict. In this area, then, the teacher, working with the child over a long span of time, can accumulate evidence seldom available from a testing situation alone.

Well defined experimental studies with young deaf children which can prove definitely that a given type of hearing problem will result in a particular kind of educational result are lacking. Nor can we say exactly which techniques of teaching will be most profitable in each particular case. Such studies are indeed much to be desired, but meanwhile, the children cannot wait. They continue to grow and to need immediate help in overcoming their hearing handicap and in learning to live in their world. Teachers must thus accept and utilize all the evidence available about each child and his hearing problem, remaining sensitive to the child's reactions and what may be learned from him as diagnostic teaching proceeds.

Let us explore some of the important differences in learning that emerge when we approach the question of hearing diagnosis from this angle.

At the Cleveland Hearing and Speech Center children ranging in age from 17 to 36 months are enrolled. Among them are a brother and sister who are the only children of two deaf parents. The boy, now three years old, and whom we shall call David, has been in the class for 18 months. He was presented with receptive language in the traditional approach for deaf children. He showed rather quickly precise ability in the formation and use of concepts. A canary in a cage was readily matched to a toy bird, either feathered or of cold celluloid, or to a picture of a robin. They all had for him some essence of "birdness." When the word was presented to him in speechreading, he applied it with equal facility to all such representations of "bird." Vocabulary, so taught, was retained readily and consistently. His teachers were soon scrambling for ways of presenting necessary repetitive stimulus material for his growing vocabulary with enough variety and spice to forestall his boredom. This child is an active, busy boy, with the usual impatience to be about his own affairs instead of attending to stipulated lessons. Nouns are by no means his chief verbal fare. Phrases and sentences, including all manner of functional modifiers and action words, are gobbled up just as eagerly. Once learned, his receptive speechreading vocabulary is retained consistently with a minimum of repeated contact. His parents, though deaf themselves, use oral communication with their children constantly, so that he lives in a speech environment.

This progress is not because of particular intellectual giftedness, for on the Merrill-Palmer performance test, his intelligence quotient was 110. His little sister is following exactly in her brother's footsteps. She is the youngest in the class by six months and has been in the program for two months. Yet she shows more precision and assurance in speechreading than any other child in class, her brother alone excepted.

These two children are, we think, "normal" children, with ears that receive a minimum of sound. It seems to be necessary only to present verbal language by a route that is open, in this case vision, to have these children learn as readily as any normal child, subject only to the limitations inherent in seeing rather than hearing speech.

For the next child in our group, we find the description of his receptive language not nearly so simple. We must, in fact, take a composite child, for no single one will illustrate all the differences we meet. If he, too, has a little sister, she will almost surely not follow in his footsteps, but present a complicated picture of her own. This boy, whom we may call Stephen, came to us ten months ago at eighteen months, an age at which deaf children are usually ready and eager to go ahead in language learning. He smiled when spoken to, waved a hand in imitation for "good-bye," and seemed in such small ways to be quite ready for the beginnings of language learning within the nursery class.

But he was not ready. It was not merely that he could not bear to have his mother leave him, even briefly. Much more, he was not ready to play independently nor to make friends with strangers. Above all, he was not ready to take direction. Described in this fashion, he does not seem to present any great differences from a normal baby his age. But compared with the previous child, he presented an entirely different kind of challenge.

When we realized our mistake, we counseled his mother, with considerable difficulty, to take him home to grow a little longer. She brought him back to us at the age of two, and we accepted him in the class, although he was still rather immature for the nursery routines, mild as they are.

Six months later, this is the picture he presents. He plays happily, and within normal developmental patterns. He likes his teachers and comes cheerfully at their bidding for small directed tasks. Sometimes he will take the toy bird to the bird cage. Often the airplane seems to him just as satisfactory. As he reaches for a requested toy, there is sometimes a light in his eyes, and he produces the appropriate object. More often, his eyes slide back and forth over his teacher's face without lighting anywhere and his hand hovers over the toys, coming up with one at random. On some days, he seems to understand several words quite precisely. On other days, the same words produce only a blank, unfocused stare.

Then there is Dean, at the same age as Stephen. His smile is more direct than Stephen's, and he can be depended upon for appropriate responses to a whole series of words for several days in a row. On other days, he seems never to have heard of any of them. The days when he is "with us," however, are noticeably increasing, and the days when he has not brought himself along are lessening.

The latter two children, we think, present an auditory problem compounded by something more than a peripheral hearing loss. Additional insight may be gained by a consideration of the development of expressive speech by these children, each so different from the other in behavior and in receptive capacity.

David's little sister, quite spontaneously, imitates the movement shapes of a word she sees, but without voice. She seldom offers such a word for communication, although this is emerging. Her brother, on the other hand, now uses his speech functionally. His voice is relaxed and pleasant, but uninflected on words, although his play vocalization shows considerable variation. After an action lesson, when his teacher has sketched the sentences, not in words but in stick figures, David can come back and "read" the picture sentences aloud: "David ran. David threw a ball." His articulation is very faulty, except for the clearly visible sounds. He can accept and make use of some mild articulation correction.

Stephen, for all practical purposes, uses no voice. He cries normally and lately has been induced to laugh aloud, sometimes. There are no pleasant vocal play sounds. There is sometimes a formless shout, usually in anger or distress.

Dean, on the other hand, laughs easily and heartily. He has developed a very few, perhaps four or five, imitative words that he will say upon request, easily, normally, with good inflection and articulation. He does not use these words for functional communication, except for the word "Mama."

The teacher must be alert to every possibility which may enhance the development of language in such children. She will thus need to be skillful in the use of amplification. Every child has a right to hear as much as he is able. If his ears do not receive sound adequately, and we can, by amplifying sound, transmit enough such sound through the ears to an adequately functioning auditory neurological system, then our way is clear. But what of the other children, those whose auditory problems have other components beyond simple lack of sensitivity to sound? If they are already receiving sound as indiscriminate noise, will amplifying this type of stimulus help the child, or only confuse him more?

It is only through study of the children that we may find the answers, which as of today we are still seeking. Deaf children, on the whole, accept and enjoy amplification. These children whose auditory problems are more complicated react in a variety of ways. Sometimes they vigorously reject amplification from the start. Sometimes they accept it for a while, then will have no more of it. Sometimes they acquiesce, but do not seem to profit from the use of a hearing aid. Sometimes their response seems to be clearly better with a hearing aid in a brief situation, but does not bear out its promise over longer use. There are also times when we feel sure that a child responds in a more relaxed and normal fashion to quiet, normal speech and learns more readily without the impact of amplification.

Our work in this area is still highly experimental. The children's responses have been too inconsistent to give us clear answers from observation alone. More subtle and discriminating means must be found to measure the effects of amplified sound with such children.

In any case, the best functional use these children can make of sound, amplified or not, is the goal that must be sought, for audition is our primary and most optimal channel for learning.

JAMES JERGER

DISCUSSION: DIAGNOSIS

THE authors who have written on the subject of diagnosis of deafness in childhood have presented new and exciting approaches to some very, very old problems.

From the standpoint of diagnostic evaluation, deaf children have always presented two unique problems: (1) They must be found *early*. (2) They must be found *accurately*.

Although the importance of early identification has been emphasized by each writer, the single area of greatest face validity, the baby's behavior in response to sound, has traditionally been viewed with some pessimissm. Investigators preoccupied with the scaling down of classical audiometric procedures from adults to children were often quick to conclude that "hearing" could not be tested below some given minimum age. The distinction between failure of the child and failure of the testing procedure has not always been clear.

Mrs. Downs has described, however, a pioneering attempt to use the controlled observation of behavior to screen, not first-graders, not pre-schoolers, but newborn babies; indeed, the entire newborn population of eight hospitals.

Early detection implies the mass testing of large numbers of very young babies, and, as Mrs. Downs has so cogently observed, this is a very inefficient process, since most newborns are not deaf. It is vitally important, therefore, that techniques suitable and feasible for mass screening be developed and expanded. The Denver people who have pointed the way are owed a great debt.

As important as early detection is *accurate* detection. Here the problem is twofold. First, children are difficult to test; and second, we are not always sure what is being tested.

It is only natural, therefore, that investigators in this area have been traditionally preoccupied with *objective* procedures— procedures that did not require the active participation and whole-hearted cooperation of the child. As Dr. Goldstein has emphasized, however, objectification of the child's role is of little avail if the end product is still based on subjective decisions by the examiner who reads the strip chart. The apparent failure of electrodermal response audiometry to live up to its early expectations, to which at least two of the previous authors have alluded, is perhaps a case in point.

The work on electroencephalic response audiometry which Dr. Goldstein has described, is one of the most exciting developments in many years, and one that holds immense promise; and, as he has emphasized, immense pitfalls.

It is important to learn what the averaged evoked potential can tell us about a child, but it is even more important to remember what it cannot tell us. There is a vast distance between the statement that "the peripheral auditory system is intact" and the statement that "hearing is normal."

Perhaps the most challenging feature of these new developments in behavioral and electrophysiologic measurement is that they are addressed to the basic tools of diagnostic evaluation, tools that in the past have been either very dull or nonexistent.

Too often in the past audiologists at least have shown a certain willingness to take great intuitive leaps not always justified by the precision of our basic tools of measurement. We have been, perhaps, a bit too willing to ascribe deviant behavioral patterns to theoretical constructs about brain activity when we did not, in fact, have tools precise enough to tell us about the child's hearing. The authors in this section have shown a healthy return to concern for the basic tools of measurement. There must be a growing realization that we cannot cross home plate until we have touched second and third base.

Dr. Bender has made an extremely important point in her observation that "the teacher working with the child over a long span of time, can accumulate evidence that is seldom available from a testing situation alone." Teachers who work with these children constitute a vast reservoir of information on the ultimate *validity* of our diagnostic judgments, a reservoir that we have not yet tapped with sufficient vigor.

Finally, Dr. Naunton and Dr. Mantell have effectively re-empha-

sized the important role played by the various medical special-
ties in the diagnostic evaluation of children, albeit there is observed a continuing note of discord. The otologist and the pediatrician are apparently still deadlocked over who shall bear over-
all responsibility for co-ordinating the many efforts being made
in the deaf child's behalf.

   We can only urge a speedy solution to this problem and hope
that the children will not suffer further in consequence.

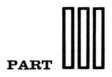

PART III

PATHOLOGY

PATHOLOGY OF SENSORINEURAL DEAFNESS OF GENETIC ORIGIN

DEAFNESS of genetic origin may be present at birth or may manifest itself in childhood or later in life. Incomplete or arrested development of the inner ear (aplasia) is a static condition. There are, however, many types of hereditary deafness which are progressive.

Environment may have a profound effect on the severity with which a genetic disorder may express itself. Heredity and environment often interact strongly, and only in extreme cases is it possible to differentiate these etiologic factors clearly. Albinism for example, is always genetic in origin, and a stab wound is always environmental. The interaction of these factors can be seen in *osteogenesis imperfecta*, where a blow could give little pathological disturbance to one individual but lead to fracture of the femur in another. The manifestations and the underlying pathology may be identical in certain disorders of genetic and environmental origin. Important factors indicating a genetic etiology are: a family history, the existence of two or more effected children in a sibship, and anatomical symmetry of the lesions (Sorsby, 1953).

Hereditary sensorineural hearing loss may be classified into the aplasias, characterized by varying degrees of incomplete development of the inner ear, the heredo-degenerations (abiotro-

Supported financially by Research Grant 05881 from the National Institutes of Health, Public Health Service.

phies) in which there is progressive loss of hearing after the inner ear has developed normally, and the chromosomal aberrations. Heredo-degenerative deafness may occur alone or in combination with other abornmalities in which case they are known as "syndromes." These syndromes are often hereditary, sometimes congenital, sometimes abiotrophic and sometimes mixed.

Genetic factors, like infectious processes, vary greatly in the severity of their effect, which is referred to as variability in "specificity". "Penetrance" is a statistical concept and refers to the frequency with which a genetic abnormality is manifested among those who possess the gene or genes involved. The severity of the disorder in a particular individual is termed "expressivity." These concepts have been well defined only in a few hereditary disorders, a good example being Waardenburg's syndrome.

Whereas these terms indicate the great variability with which an inherited disorder may express itself in succeeding generations, many investigators in studying inherited deafness have described dominant and recessive types. A character is dominant if the manifestation of the defect is linked to the presence of a gene on only one chromosome of a given chromosome pair. A recessive gene, on the other hand, produces its effect only if it is present on both elements of a chromosome pair and remains unexpressed if it is present only on one chromosome.

Sex-linked types of deafness have also been described. This is caused by the fact that the sex chromosomes carry, not only the factors for determination of sex and secondary sexual characteristics, but in addition a number of characters that have nothing to do with sex.

Chromosomal aberrations are responsible for a number of severe anomalies. The presence of an extra chromosome (trisomy) leads to anomalies associated with deafness. The most common are Trisomy 13 and Trisomy 18. Whereas most chromosomal aberrations are probably due to mutations, it is well established that translocation of a chromosome or part of a chromosome may occur as a familial trait transmitted by the mother and results in a higher incidence of the trisomy syndrome in the offspring.

The following classification of sensorineural deafness of genetic origin is based on a study of the literature and the temporal bone specimens from several laboratories. The Bing-Siebenmann classification of aplasia, described by Ormerod (1960) and others seems too vague and too poorly documented to be included as an entity at this time. It has been characterized as consisting of a well formed, bony labyrinth, but an underdeveloped membranous part, particularly the sense organs. Also, the Siebenmann type of aplasia has been omitted. It is said to consist mainly of changes in the middle ear due to hormone deficiency, as typified by the cretin anomalies. The following classification provides no information, of course, on the incidence of the various types of hereditary deafness. The aplasias and the trisomy types are relatively infrequent compared with the heredo-degenerations.

Classifications for Deafness of Genetic Origin

A. The *Aplasias*

    1. Michel: complete failure of development of the inner ear.

    2. Mondini: incomplete development of bony and membranous labyrinth.

    3. Scheibe: membranous cochleo-saccular aplasia.

    4. Alexander: membranous cochlear aplasia.

        a. basal turn, high-frequency loss, descending audiometric pattern.

        b. all turns, all frequencies, basin type audiometric pattern.

B. The *Heredo-degenerations*

    1. Occurring alone

        a. Infantile

        b. Adult

    2. Associated with other abnormalities

        a. essentially mesodermal
        e.g. Gargoylism, Marfan's, chondrodystrophy, Alport's, Pendred's, Jervell's.

        b. essentially ectodermal
        e.g. Waardenburg's, Usher's

        c. essentially neuroectodermal
        e.g. Recklinghausen's neurofibromatosis, the cerebellar degenerations.

C. *Chromosomal Aberrations*

    1. Trisomy 13 (D_1)

    2. Trisomy 18 (E)

Aplasia of the Inner Ear

Aplasia of the inner ear implies failure of complete development. It is always congenital; that is, it is always present at birth. The various types, based on the degree of development, have been described by Ormerod (1960) and others. Individual cases may not fall specifically into one type or another and the classification must be considered in the broad sense. The time at which development was arrested determines the ultimate structural appearance of the ear. An individual may possess different degrees of aplasia in the two ears. The Sheibe type (cochleo-saccular aplasia) is the most common with the Mondini (aplasia of bony and membranous labyrinth) next in order of frequency. The Michel type (total failure of development of the inner ear) is rare.

Michel: Complete Failure of Development of the Inner Ear (*Michel*, 1863).

In some cases, the petrous portion of the temporal bone fails to develop; in others it is present but underdeveloped at the normal location of the labyrinth. In some cases, there may be spaces in the bone which do not resemble inner-ear structure. The external and middle ears may be normal. In Michel's original case, the malleus, incus, and tensor tympani muscle were normal, but the stapes was missing.

Ear 1, Infant T. (Reported by Jorgensen, et al., 1964). During the gestation period, the mother of this infant was administered 1 or 2 tablets containing Thalidomide about 25 days after conception. Labor was induced ten days beyond the calculated term and the baby was anoxic at the time of birth. Radiography revealed severe aplasia of the middle and inner ears on both sides. At the age of four months the infant died. Autopsy revealed an aterial septal defect four cm. in size. There was no evidence of an internal auditory meatus on either side.

Histological examination showed a small middle ear and ossicles on both sides. On the left side there was a labyrinthine bony capsule with a small inner ear space without an organized membranous labyrinth.

On the right side (see Figure 1), there was no evidence of an inner ear, and the auditory, vestibular, and facial nerves were absent. This right ear belongs to the rare Michel type, that is, total aplasia of the inner ear.

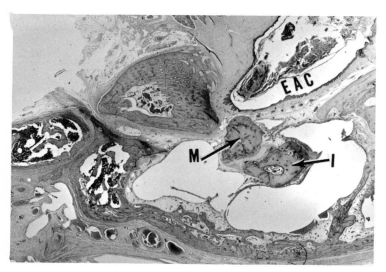

Figure 1. Ear 1, Infant T, courtesy of H. K. Kristensen, Copenhagen, Michel-type inner-ear aplasia caused by Thalidomide. The external auditory canal (EAC), the malleus (M), and the incus (I) are normal. The labyrinth is missing completely.

Mondini: Incomplete Development of the Bony and Membranous Labyrinth (Mondini, 1791).

This condition has been described as consisting of a flattened cochlea with development of only the basal turn associated with a similar degree of underdevelopment of the labyrinth at about the sixth week of gestation. The canals are often unformed but may be represented by discs of compact bone without a lumen. In some cases, there may be some cochlear or vestibular sensory epithelium. Often there is underdevelopment in the opposite ear of a different degree.

Ear 2, Child M. C. (Reported by J. S. Fraser, 1926, 1927). This was the twelfth child of healthy parents. Soon after birth he appeared to have mild hydrocephalis. He turned his head to the right and had to be propped up in his perambulator. His motor development was slow and he appeared to be mentally retarded. He did not speak, but made inarticulate noises. At the age of five it was determined that he could hear a whistle. He died suddenly during a tonsillectomy and the temporal bones were removed for study.

Histological examination showed a severe degree of aplasia of both inner ears, more marked on the left side.

Fraser's description of the right ear may be summarized as follows: The bony cochlea is somewhat flattened from base to apex and the modiolus is badly formed, consisting of only 1½ turns. The cochlear duct of the upper part of the basal turn is very small and the vestibule is very wide. The spiral ganglion cell population to the existing basal turn is slightly diminished. The tectorial membrane appears club-shaped in some areas and does not make contact with the organ of Corti. The utricle is large but the neural epithelium of the macule is poorly developed. The saccule is normal. The horizontal semicircular canal is small, but the other two canals are normal. Both the cochlear and vestibular nerves are well developed. (Figure 2)

Scheibe: Cochleosaccular Aplasia (Scheibe, 1891, 1892).

In this type of aplasia, the bony labyrinth is fully developed and the aplasia involves only the phylogenetically newer part of the

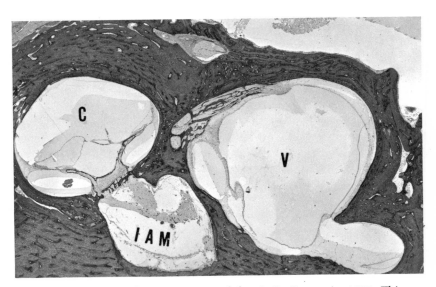

Figure 2. Ear 2, Child M. D., reported by J. S. Fraser in 1927. This ear represents the Mondini-type aplasia, that is, aplasia of both the bony and membranous labyrinths. The cochlea (C) consists of only 1½ turns instead of 2½. The vestibule (V) contains a large deformed utricle. The internal auditory meatus (IAM) contains normal appearing cochlear, vestibular, and facial nerves.

inner ear, that is, the cochlea and the saccule. The utricle and canals are histologically normal and function normally. There are characteristic changes of the stria vascularis consisting of areas of aplasia alternating with regions of hyperplasia and gross deformity. Reissner's membrane is usually collapsed and lying on the stria and on the rudimentary sense organ. The tectorial membrane often has a rounded appearance and lies in the internal sulcus. The supporting elements of the organ of Corti are distorted and collapsed, and only an occasional hair cell can be identified. The appearance is almost identical to that seen in inherited deafness in some animals, such as Dalmation dogs.

The wall of the saccule is depressed and lying on the atrophic sensory epithelium and the deformed otolithic membrane. Usually the spiral ganglion is normal and may remain so until late in life.

Ear 3, Infant F. (Specimen From the Laboratory of Prof. L. Ruedi). This full-term infant died ten hours after birth of asphyxiation. The father and mother were known to be "deaf-mutes."

Histological examination of the right ear reveals a normally developed external auditory canal, middle ear, internal auditory meatus and bony capsule. There is aplasia of the structures in the cochlear duct and the saccule. The utricle and semicircular canals appear normal.

The stria vascularis is atrophic in some areas and hyperplastic in others. In some areas it forms multiple layers separated by fibrous tissue, protruding into the cochlear duct and adherent to a collapsed Reissner's membrane. Reissner's membrane is depressed toward the basilar membrane throughout, reducing the size of the endolymphatic space to one half or less of normal. There is moderately severe postmortem autolysis of the organ of Corti, however, some hair cells can be identified. The tectorial membrane has a rounded shape and is lying in the internal sulcus. The population of spiral ganglion cells is normal.

The saccular wall is collapsed and lying on an irregular distorted otolithic membrane and the sensory epithelium appears atrophic (Figures 3 and 4).

Alexander: Membranous Cochlear Aplasia (Alexander 1927).

In 1927, Alexander described congenital familial nonprogressive high tone sensorineural deafness, which has subsequently been recognized as a hereditary entity. This is well demonstrated in the

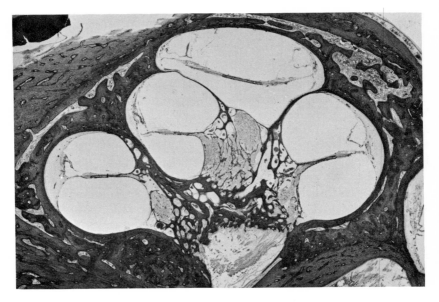

Figure 3. Ear 3, Infant F., courtesy of Professor L. Ruedi, Zurich. Scheibe-type aplasia (cochleo-saccular) in a newborn whose parents were known to be "deaf-mutes." The structures of the cochlear duct are underdeveloped and deformed. The spiral ganglion is normal.

family whose audiograms appear in Figure 5. A pedigree has not been established for this family, and it is possible that the deafness is sex-linked, as all afflicted members are females.

Another variation of the Alexander type of partial cochlear aplasia are those individuals with a mid-frequency hearing loss, characterized by the "basin-shaped" audiometric pattern. These individuals have unusually good speech discrimination scores, indicating an excellent nerve in the cochlea.

The Heredo-degenerations (abiotrophies)

Hereditary Progressive Deafness Occurring Alone

Goodhill (1950) has classified this acquired hereditary type of deafness into infantile and adult types, however, Cawthorne and Hinchcliffe (1957) found a continuous distribution of the age of onset. Albrecht (1923) showed that familial progressive nerve deafness is transmitted by a dominant gene, and Johnson (1952) confirmed this. Ford (1952) described two families with progres-

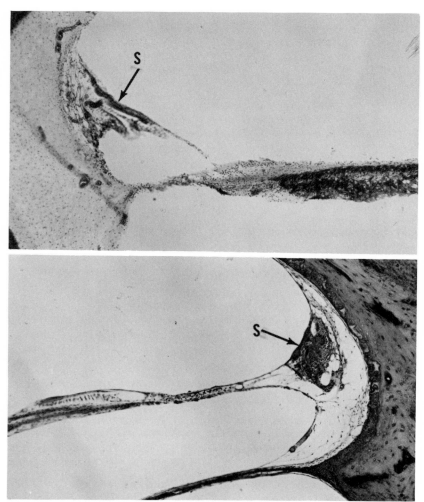

Figure 4. Views of the cochlear duct of Infant F (Figure 3) and Infant N (also born deaf) showing the characteristic deformity of the stria (S) in the Scheibe-type aplasia.

sive nerve deafness due to recessive inheritance and Ersner and Saltzman (1941) reported a family with sex-linked recessive inherited deafness.

The audiometric patterns may vary considerably, but most commonly are more severe for high frequencies, being of either

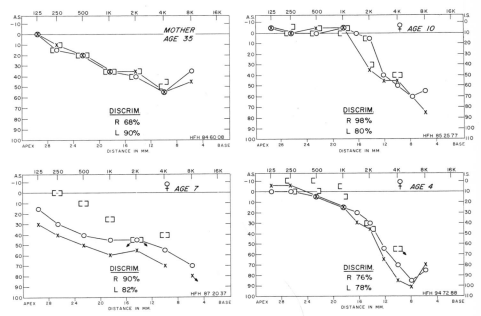

Figure 5. Audiograms of mother and three daughters, all with high-tone hearing losses which were present at birth, apparently not progressive or only slightly progressive, and possibly sex-linked. There are no male siblings. The 7-year-old had serous otitis media at the time of the test which subsequently disappeared. The hereditary deafness in this family represents the Alexander-type of cochlear aplasia.

the abrupt or gradual descending types. The pathological correlate is a degenerative change in the sensory and neural elements of the basal turn.

Another type of heredo-degenerative deafness which is less well documented is characterized by a flat audiometric pattern with excellent speech discrimination and is caused by degeneration of the stria vascularis.

Associated with Other Abnormalities (The Syndromes).

These syndromes, characterized as clinical entities, involving several organs and manifested by degenerative changes, have little or no relationship to each other. The entities cannot be explained on the basis of metabolic, embryologic, or infectious pathogenesis, but are more comprehensible in the terms of genetics. It seems pathogentically useful to classify the syndromes into essentially mesodermal syndromes, ectodermal syndromes and neuro-ectodermal syndromes, according to the suggestion of Francois (1961).

Mesodermal Syndromes.—These syndromes consist of varying, but generally consistent patterns of mesodermal disorders associated with deafness. Following are several examples well known to otology:

Gargoylism (Hurler's Syndrome). Hurler (1919) first fully described this disorder, also known as gargoylism, recognizing it as a hereditary disease, and considering it to be a primary skeletal growth disturbance. Classically, the disease begins in early childhood, causing skeletal deformity, failure of mental development, blindness, enlargement of the liver and spleen, and sometimes deafness. The disorder is probably hereditary of the recessive type.

Marfan's Syndrome (Marfan 1896) usually consists of a number of congenital anomalies among which may be found:

Arachnodactyle (possibly also scoliosis, pigeon breast, flat feet, hammer toe, doliocephaly, and high arched palate)

Ectopia lentis (dislocation of the lens)

Deafness, sensorineural or conductive or both

Hypotonic muscles and laxity of joints, ligaments, and cartilage

Anomalies of the heart and lungs

The hearing loss may be of the conductive type due to meso-dermal anomalies characterized by large soft auricles without cartilaginous support with abnormal configuration (Ganther, 1927; Everberg, 1959). Others have reported an associated sensorineural type deafness (Brock, 1929; Schilling, 1936).

Chondrodystrophy. Chondrodystrophy is a hereditary skeletal disease transmitted as a simple dominant mendalian factor (Keizer and Schilder, 1951, Caffey and Ross, 1958). As a result of defective growth and maturation of cartilage, the bones of the extremities are short and thick. Similar changes occur in the base of the skull which lead to reduction in length of the cranial base, deep saddling of the nose, and relative protrusions of the mandible and frontal bones. These are the achondroplastic dwarfs of the circus. They possess normal intelligence and show no evidence of glandular dysfunction. Although many die at birth or shortly thereafter, others may live to become adults and to propagate the inherited traits. Deafness is frequently present and often is combined conductive and sensorineural in type.

Ear 4, Infant C. (Specimen From the Laboratory of Prof. L. Ruedi). Histological examination of two horizontal sections of this infant's temporal bone reveal that the membranous labyrinth is encased in a layer of normal-appearing endosteal bone. The enchondral and periosteal bone has dense thick trabeculae without islands of cartilage. There is very spare cellularity of the intertrabecular spaces.

The bony cochlear canals are deformed and the intercochlear partitions are thickened. The membranous labyrinth has undergone severe postmortem autolysis, and the sense organs cannot be evaluated histologically. The spiral ganglion cell population appears normal. (Figure 6)

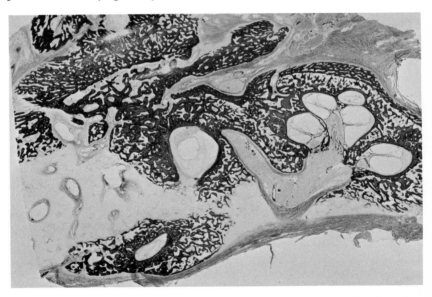

Figure 6. Ear 4, Infant C., courtesy of Professor L. Ruedi, Zurich. Chrondrodysplasia in a newborn characterized by absence of cartilage in the enchondral layer and deformity of the bony labyrinth.

Pendred's Syndrome. Pendred (1896) presented the findings in two sisters with profound sensorineural deafness and large goiters. The deafness had been present since infancy, and the goiters were first noted at about the age of thirteen. One sister was mentally deficient and the other intelligent. Both had normal body builds. Brain (1927) reported on twelve individuals with deafness from the time of birth and goiters occurring in middle childhood. Deraemaker (1956) Thieme (1957) and Elman (1958) describe similar findings in single families. Fraser, et al. (1961) reported the findings in 113 cases from 72 families. The syndrome is characterized by the following features: sensorineural hearing loss existing at birth; goiter usually occurring during childhood or adolescence.

Schools for the deaf contain many of these individuals.

Jervell's Syndrome. Jervell, et al. (1957) reported a syndrome observed in four children of a family of six in Scandinavia. The syndrome has the following features: sensorineural deafness, present at birth; syncopal attacks; prolonged Q-T interval in the EKG; sudden death early in life.

Alport's Syndrome. Dickinson (1875) referred to three generations of a family in which 11 of the 17 members had albuminuria and several died prematurely of nephritis. This is apparently the first report in the literature of hereditary renal disease, and no mention was made of associated deafness.

It was Alport (1927) who pointed out the high incidence of sensorineural deafness in those individuals afflicted with "hereditary, familial, congenital, hemorrhagic nephritis."

Ectodermal Syndromes. The ectodermal syndromes consist mainly of disorders of the auditory and visual sense organs along with pigmentary changes.

Waardenburg's Syndrome. Waardenburg (1951) first described a new syndrome consisting of lateral displacement of the medial canthae and lacrimal puncta; a hyperplastic high nasal root; hyperplasia of the medial portions of the eyebrows; partial or total heterochromia iridium; sensorineural deafness, bilateral or unilateral: circumscribed albinism of the frontal head hair (white forelock).

There are several other syndromes in which deafness is associated with ectodermal dysplasias, particularly pigmentary alterations. Among these are piebaldness, albinism, and *pili torti* (Fragile twisted hair).

Usher's Syndrome. A survey of the literature reveals that von Graefe (1858) was the first to describe this syndrome, but it is usually termed Usher's syndrome because of his more extensive study of this disorder (Usher, 1914). Characteristic features of this syndrome may be listed as follows: retinitis pigmentosa; sensorineural type deafness; vestibulo-cerebellar ataxia; mental disorder.

Neuroectodermal Syndromes. Forms of deafness associated with disease of the central nervous system have been listed by Kluyskens and Geldof (1965) as follows: cerebral palsy, the juvenile form of leucodystrophy, the juvenile form of cerebellar degeneration (Schilder's syndrome), polyganglioradicular heredopathia, and hypertrophic neuritis of Dejerine-Sottas.

Recklinghausen's neurofibromatosis may be present at birth, appear in childhood, or late in life. It is characterized by a triad of symptoms: Subcutaneous tumors, nerve tumors (schwannomas) and pigmentary changes. Deafness is frequent and may be unilateral or bilateral, of the sensorineural type, caused by schwannomas in the internal auditory meatus.

Chromosomal Aberrations

The discovery of an extra chromosome as the cause of mongoloidism by Lejeune, *et al.* (1959) and by Jacobs *et al.* (1959), initiated studies in a new field of genetics. DeWolff (1963) studied the chromosomal patterns in monovular twins, one of which was mongoloid. The mongoloid child had an additional chromosome 21 which carried the same genes as one of the other two chromosomes of the same number. Thus, a new genetic principle was established—that the normal number of genes must be present in balanced number to produce a normal zygote. Deviations from the normal number may lead to serious alterations of the phenotype.

Trisomy 13 (D₁). Infants afflicted with this syndrome fail to thrive, and most die within a few weeks or months. The ear, nose, and throat findings in 36 cases of Trisomy D reported by Zellwager (1965) are as follows:

Trisomy D

Low-set ears	12
Poorly differentiated pinnae	17
Pre-auricular tags	3
Absence of external auditory canal	4
Absence of middle ear	1
Cleft lip and/or palate	21
Micrognathia	5
Microphthalmia	13
Iris coloboma	11
Cataracts	9
Retrolental membrane	4
Anophthalmia	4
Retinaldysplasia	3
Hypoplasia or aplasia of optic nerve	12
Facial capillary hemangioma	13

Ear 5, Infant C. M.—Trisomy 13–15. This full-term, white female was born to a 41-year-old mother and a 42-year-old father. There is a history of previous miscarriages. Birth weight was 7 lbs., 2 oz. (3.2 kg.). The infant presented multiple anomalies, consisting of microcephaly, complete cleft palate and harelip, failure of mesial growth of the parietal bones with scalp defect, microphthalmia, bilateral, colobomata, low-set, malformed ears, polydactyly, seizures, and failure to respond to sound. The clinical appearance suggested 13–15 trisomy syndrome, which was confirmed by chromosomal studies. The child died at the age of 25 days. Right and left temporal bones were obtained for pathological study.

The histopathological findings in both ears were similar and may be described together. The external auditory canal, tympanic membrane, and other middle-ear structures appear normal. The mastoid shows normal development for this infant.

The inner-ear changes are limited to the cochlea and saccule. In the basal turn, the organ of Corti is either missing or replaced by a layer of fibrous tissue (Figure 7). In the middle and apical turns, some of the supporting cells of the organ of Corti are present, but hair cells are missing. The tectorial membrane lies in the inner sulcus and is encapsulated by a single layer of cells. Reissner's membrane is completely missing in the lower basal

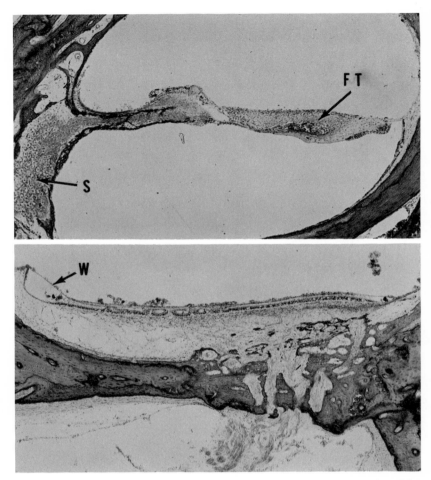

Figure 7. Ear 5, Infant C. M., Trisomy 13. The organ of Corti is replaced by a thick layer of fibrous tissue (F. T.), in the basal turn, although the spiral ganglion (S) is normal. The saccular wall (W) is collapsed onto the macula. The sensory epithelium of the macula is disorganized and missing in some areas.

turn and is atrophic and in contact with the organ of Corti and stria vascularis in the remainder of the cochlea. The stria vascularis is atrophied or missing in the lower basal turn. The spiral ganglion is normal throughout.

The saccular wall is collapsed and lying upon the macula. The sensory epithelium of the macule of the saccule is disorganized and missing in some areas. The otolithic membrane can be identified as a thin layer of homogeneous material without evidence of statoconia. There are some cystic areas in the sensory epithelium. The saccular nerve appears normal.

The utricle and the semicircular canals are normal.

Trisomy 18 (E). The incidence of ear, nose and throat findings in 67 cases of Trisomy E observed by Zellweger (1965) are as follows:

Trisomy E

Low-set ears	62
Poorly differentiated pinnae	54
Micrognathia	58
High palate	22
Cleft lip and/or palate	7
Ptosis of eyelids	10
Absence of external auditory canal, microstomia, choanal atresia, slanting eyes, microphthalmia, iris coloboma, glaucoma, optic atrophy	Rare

Ear 6, Infant P. N.—Trisomy 18. This white male was the product of the sixth pregnancy of a 38-year-old mother and a 41-year-old father. Birth weight was 5 lbs. (3.1 kg.). Physical findings included bilateral inquinal hernias, prominent occiput, micrognathia, high-arched palate, low-set pointed ears, typical hand posture, and rocker-bottom feet. The infant responded to loud sounds. Chromosome analysis confirmed the clinical diagnosis of 18 trisomy syndrome. The patient died at the age of $3^1/2$ months. Both temporal bones were obtained for pathological study.

Histological examination of the right ear revealed the malleus and incus to be slightly deformed but the ossicular joints to be normal. The tensor tympani muscle has an unusual anatomical course in that its fibers are divided into two bundles in separate bony canals. The fibers which are most lateral follow the normal pathway toward the cochleariform process, and the fibers which are located medially go to an aberrant canal to join the facial nerve in the fallopian canal. Superior to the stapes footplate this latter bundle leaves the facial canal and attaches par-

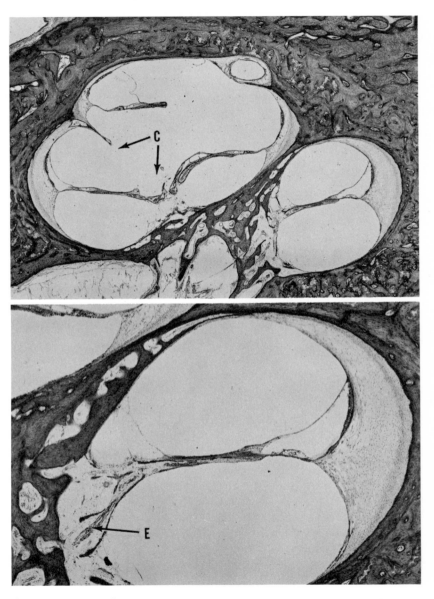

Figure 8. Ear 6, Infant P. N., Trisomy 18. Scala communis (C) exists between the middle and apical turns. Rosenthal's canal is very small, and only a few spiral ganglion cells are present in the basal turn only. The nerve fibers which are present apparently are efferents (E).

tially to the wall of the sinus tympani and ends by joining the fibers of the stapedial muscle.

The mastoid appears normal for an infant of this age.

The bony modiolus is incompletely developed. Some of the spiral ganglion cells lie in the internal auditory meatus. The population of spiral ganglion cells appears normal. The organ of Corti, the saccular and utricular maculae, and the cristae appear normal. The vestibular nerves are normal.

Histological examination of the left ear showed the cochlea to be somewhat flattened and the bony partition between the middle and apical turns to be partially missing (scala communis).

There is almost complete absence of the spiral ganglion. Only a few ganglion cells remain in Rosenthal's canal at the extreme basal end of the cochlea. There are small bundles of nerve fibers which enter the modiolus and pass to the organ of Corti throughout the cochlea which probably represent the efferent fibers of the olivocochlear bundle. The hair-cell population of the organ of Corti appears normal. The stria vascularis is incompletely developed (Figure 8). The saccule, utricle, and semicircular canals appear normal. Scarpa's ganglia and the fibers of the vestibular nerves appear normal.

Summary

Sensorineural deafness of genetic origin may be characterized by incomplete development of the inner ear (aplasias), progressive degeneration of the inner ear (heredo-degenerative abiotrophies) and chromosomal aberrations (trisomies). The apasias and chromosomal anomalies are relatively uncommon. The heredo-degenerative types of deafness are common and may occur alone or in combination with other abnormalities when they are known as syndromes. These syndromes may be classified as mesodermal, ectodermal, and neuroectodermal, according to the combination of anomalies which are present.

References

Albrecht, W. 1923. "Ueber die Vererbung der konstitutionell sporadischen Taubstummheit, der hereditaren Labyrinthschwerhörigkeit und der Otosclerose." Arch. f. Ohrenheilk, 110:15–48.

Alexander, G. 1927. "Die Ohrenkrankheiten im Kindesalter." C. W. Vogel, pp. 24, 171.

Alport, A. C. 1927. "Hereditary Familiar Congenital Haemorrhagic Nephritis." *Brit. M. J.*, **1**(March 19):504–506.

Brain, W. R. 1927. "Heredity in Simple Goitre." *Quart. J. Med.*, **20** (April):303–319.

Brock, J. 1929. "Weiterer Beitrag zur Lehre von der Arachnodaktylie." *Ztschr. Kinderh.* **47**:702–714.

Caffey, J., and S. Ross. 1958. "Pelvic Bones in Infantile Mongoloidism; Roentenographic Features." *Am. J. Roentgenol.*, **80**(Sept.):458–467.

Cawthorne, T. E., and R. Hinchcliffe. 1957. "Familial Perceptive Deafness. *Pract. oto-rhino-laryng.*, **19**:69–83.

Deraemaeker, R. 1956. "Congenital Deafness and Goiter." *Am. J. Human Genet.*, **8**(Dec.)253–256.

de Wolff, E., K. Schärrer, and J. Lejeune. 1962. ("Contribution à l'étude des jumeaux mongoliens: un cas de monozygotisme hétércaryote.") *Helvet. paediat. acta*, **17**:301–328.

Dickinson, W. H. 1875. *Diseases of the Kidney, Pt. I.* London: Longmans, Green & Co. P. 379.

Elman, D. S. 1958. "Familial Association of Nerve Deafness With Nodular Goiter and Thyroid Carcinoma." *New England J. Med.*, **259** (July 31):219–223.

Ernsner, M. S., and M. Saltzman. 1941. "Progressive Analogous Nerve Deafness in Three Successive Generations With Sex-Limited Inheritance." *Laryngoscope*, **51**(March):41–245.

Everberg, G. 1959. "Marfan's Syndrome Associated With Hearing Defect: Report of a Case in One of a Pair of Twins." *Acta paediat.*, **48**(Jan.):70–76.

Ford, F. D. 1952. *Diseases of the Nervous System in Infancy, Childhood and Adolescence.* Springfield, Illinois: Thomas.

Francois, J. 1961. *Heredity in Ophthalmology.* St. Louis, Missouri: Mosby.

Fraser, G. R., M. E. Morgans, and W. R. Trotter. 1961. "Sporadic Goitre With Congenital Deafness (Pendred's Syndrome)." *Advances in Thyroid Research, Transactions of the Fourth International Goitre Conference, London, July 1960,* edited by R. Pitt-Rivers. Oxford: Pergamon Press, P. 19.

Fraser, J. S. 1926–1927. "A Case of Congenital Deafness With Malformation of the Membranous Labyrinthis of Both Sides." *Proc. Roy. Soc. Med. Sect. Otol.*, **20**:17–19. *J. Laryng. & Otol.*, **42**(May):315–321.

Ganther, R. 1927. "Ein Beitrag zur Arachnodaktylie." *Ztschr. Kinderh.*, **43**:724–736.

Goodhill, V. 1950. "The Nerve-Deaf Child: Significance of Rh, Maternal Rubella and Other Etiologic Factors." *Ann. Otol. Rhin. & Laryng.* **59**(Dec.):1123–1147.

Hurler, G. 1920. "Ueber einen Typ Multipler Abartgungen, vorwiegend am Skelettsystem." *Ztsch. Kinderh.*, **24**:220–34.

Jacobs, P. A., A. G. Baikie, W. M. Court Brown, and J. A. Strong. 1959. "The Somatic Chromosomes in Mongolism." *Lancet*, **1**(April 4):710.

Jervell, A., and F. Lange-Nielsen. 1957. "Congenital Deaf-Mutism, Functional Heart-Disease With Prolongation of the Q-T Interval and Sudden Death." *Am. Heart. J.*, **54**(July):59–68.

Johnson, S. 1952. "The Heredity of Perceptive Deafness." *Acta otolaryng.*, **42**:539–552.

Jorgensen, M. B., H. K. Kristensen, and N. H. Buch. 1964. "Thalidomide-Induced Aplasia of the Inner Ear." *J. Laryng. & Otol.*, **78**(Dec.):1095–1101.

Keizer, D. P. R., and J. N. Schilder. 1951. "Ectodermal Dysplasia, Achondrodysplasia, and Congenital Morbus Cordis." *Amer. J. Dis. Child,* **82**(Sept.):341–344.

Kluyskens, P., and H. Geldof. 1965. "La surdité héréditaire." *Acta ocorhino-laryng. belg.*, **19**:519–543.

Lejeune, J., M. Gautier, and R. Turpin. 1959. "Étude des chromosomes somatiques de neur enfants mongoliens." *Compt. rend. Acad. sc.*, **248**(March 16):1721–1722.

Marfan, A. B. 1896. "Un cas de déformation congénitale des quatre membres, plus pronouncée aux entrémités, caracterisée par l'allongement des os avec un certain degré d'amincissement." *Bull. et mém, Soc. méd. hôp. Paris*, **13**:220–226.

Michel, E. M. 1863. "Mémoire sur les anomalies congenitales de l'oreille interne." *Gaz. Méd. Strasb.*, **3**:55–58.

Mondini, C. 1791. "Anatomia surdi nedi sectio." *De Bononiensi Scientiarum et Artium Instituto Atque Academi Commentarii, Bologna*, **7**:28–29, 419–431.

Ormerod, F. C. 1960. "Pathology of Congenital Deafness." *J. Laryng. & Otol.*, **74**(Dec.)919–950.

Pendred, V. 1896. "Deaf-Mutism and Goitre." *Lancet*, **2**:532.

Scheibe, A. 1891–1892. "Ein fall von Taubstummheit mit Acusticusatrophie und Bildungsanomalien im häutigen Labyrinth beiderseits." *Ztsch. Ohrenh.*, **22**:11–23.

Scheibe, A. 1892. "A Case of Deaf-Mutism, With Auditory Atrophy and Anomalies of Development in the Membranous Labyrinth of Both Ears. *Arch. Otol.*, **21**:12–22.

Schilling, V. 1936. "Striae distensae als hypophysäris Symptom bei basophilen Vorderlappenadenom und bei Arachnodaktylie mit Hypophysentumor. *Med. Welt.*, **10**(Feb. 8):183; **10**(Feb. 15):219; **10**(Feb. 22):259.

Sorsby, A. 953. *Clinical Genetics.* St. Louis, Missouri: Mosby.

Thieme, E. T. (1957). "A Report of the Occurrence of Deaf-Mutism and Goiter in Four of Six Siblings of a North American Family." *Ann. Surg.*, **146**(Dec.):941–948.

Usher, C. H. 1914. "On the Inheritance of Retinitis Pigmentosa, with Notes of a Case." *Roy. London Ophth. Hosp. Rep.*, **19**:130–236.

v. Graefe, A. 1858. "Vereinzelte Beobatchtungen und Bemerkunge. No. 6. Exceptionelles Verhalten des Gesichsfeldes bei Pigmentenartung der Netzhaut." *Arch. f. Ophth.*, **4**:250–253.

Waardenburg, P. J. 1951. "A New Syndrome Combining Developmental Anomalies of the Eyelids, Eyebrows, and Nose Root with Pigmentary Defects of the Iris and Head Hair and With Congenital Deafness." *Am. J. Human Genet.*, **3**(Sept.):195–253.

Zellweger, H. 1965. "Chromosomal Aberrations and Their Significance for Ophthalmo-Otorhinolaryngology." *Tr. Am. Acad. Ophth.*, **69**(Jan.-Feb.):33–50.

THE PATHOLOGY OF ACQUIRED VIRAL ENDOLABYRINTHITIS

FOR many years viruses have been recognized as a cause of acquired nerve deafness.

Among viruses known or suspected to cause deafness are mumps, measles, chickenpox, influenza, common cold viruses, and poliomyelitis (Bordley and Hardy, 1951; Zonderman, B, 1959; Shambaugh, et al., 1928; Yearsley, 1934; Kinney, 1953; Whetnall and Fry, 1964). Virus disease is considered, mainly on clinical grounds, to be the etiology of some cases of sudden deafness with or without vertigo. (Lindsay and Zuidema, 1950; Lindsay, 1959; Schuknecht, et al., 1962; Saunders and Lippy, 1959). Ward, et al. (1965) described cytomegalic inclusion disease affecting the endothelium of the small blood vessels of the petrous apex in a 48-year-old woman who died of irreversible shock following a colectomy for ulcerative colitis. This virus has not yet however been implicated as a cause of inner-ear pathology.

A virus is a unique and different type of infectious agent in that it has a relatively simple chemical composition, is smaller than other infectious agents, lacks enzymes for energy metabolism, and appears to have no life of its own outside of cells and multiplies intracellularly.

Viral protein is antigenic and its nucleic acid is different from that of the host cells in which it is synthesized. The nucleic acid is the genetic material of the virus and accounts for the transmission of heritable characters during virus multiplication. Viruses apparently cause infected cells to produce new materials and

91

develop properties different from those of normal cells and may cause cells to respond in one of the following ways: degeneration and death, neoplastic transformation, and survival without transformation but with evidence of viral presence.

A virus contains either ribonucleic or deoxyribonucleic acid. No virus has both types of nucleic acid. Virus groups are listed in Table I (after Horstall and Tamm, 1965).

TABLE I

CLASSES OF VIRUSES

RNA Viruses	Example	DNA Viruses	Example
Picornavirus	Poliovirus Coxsackie virus	Papovavirus	Various wart viruses
Reovirus	Types I, II, III	Adenovirus	Viruses causing acute respiratory disease Viruses causing conjunctivitis
Arbovirus	Western equine encephalitis virus Yellow fever virus	Herpesvirus	Herpes simplex Cytomelagoviruses
Myxovirus	Measles, Mumps	Poxvirus	Smallpox (Variola) Vaccinia virus

The Measles Virus

The measles virus is classified under the myxoviruses. The virus is a roughly ovoid or spherical particle 120 to 250 millimicrons in diameter. It contains an inner helix about 170 angstroms in diameter which is probably composed of ribonucleoprotein and ribonucleic acid. Surrounding the helix is a lipoprotein envelope. Protruding from this envelope are multiple spikes which are thought to contain some of the antigenic substances. All measles strains appear to be antigenically homogeneous. In the lipoprotein envelope are found hemolyzing, hemagglutinating, and some of the complement fixing antigens. Measles virus has certain antigens in common with canine distemper and bovine rinderpest, but these do not cause problems in serodiagnosis of measles because man is resistant to rinderpest, and canine distemper does not yield antibodies capable of reacting with measles virus. The hemagglutination-inhibition test is used to detect measles antibody (Waterson, et al., 1961; Horsfall and Tamm, 1965).

General Clinical Picture

The two-to-four-day prodromal period of measles infection is characterized by fever and increasing respiratory symptoms. The enanthem or Koplik spot then appears—a small, irregular, bright red spot with a tiny, bluish-white center. Conjunctival inflammation also appears. Viremia is present during the prodrome, and respiratory secretions yield large amounts of virus. The measles virus has been found in many tissues in patients dying during the prodromal phase.

The characteristic rash or exanthem then appears, spreading downward from the scalp line. The lesions are macular or maculopapular, often confluent or blotchy and blanch on pressure. The rash and fever gradually resolve in four to five days, the rash leaving behind a brown stain, followed by branny desquamation. The rash may be hemorrhagic and may be associated with visceral hemorrhage which may be fatal (Kempe and Fulginiti, 1965; Horsfall and Tamm, 1965).

Pathogenesis and Pathology

Measles virus is probably deposited primarily onto the upper respiratory mucosa and into the conjunctival sac, but whether primary multiplication occurs there is not known. Viremia is found on the fifth to seventh day after experimental introduction of virus in monkeys. Evidence indicates that the virus multiplies in the reticuloendothelial tissue before this, possibly after an early, as yet undemonstrated viremia. The virus is found in the circulating white cells, and a leukopenia is present. Possibly the virus multiplies in the white cells which are then lysed by an unknown mechanism, releasing virus into the blood stream. Chromosome breakage is found in the white cells.

The early pathology of human measles is largely unknown. In monkeys within three days following incubation some generalized lymphoid hyperplasia and giant-cell formation is seen. Epithelial and lymphoid giant cells have been seen in the nasal secretions, vermiform appendix and other lymphoid tissue of human patients. The lymphoid giant cells are called Warthin-Finkeldey cells and may be up to 100 microns in diameter and may contain up to 100 nuclei. The Koplik spot consists of focal exudations of serum and endothelial cells in the form of vesicles which become necrotic. The skin rash starts with exudation of serum and proliferation of endothelial cells around the superficial vessels of the corium. The exudate spreads into the epidermis; vacuoles, necrosis of the epithelial eclls, and vesicles form. Lymphocytes infiltrate perivascularly; occasionally red blood cells are extravasated. If encephalitis ensues, congestion and petechial hemorrhages are seen in the brain. Microscopically there is an early perivascular hemorrhage and lymphocytic infiltration; later demyelinated areas, which may have some leukocytic infiltrates and gliosis, appear (Kempe and Fulginiti, 1965; Horsfall and Tamm, 1965).

Measles virus is known to cross the placental barrier, as infants born of mothers with measles have also shown the disease (Dyer, 1940; Packer, 1950.). Measles early in pregnancy may cause spontaneous abortion, may be compatible with survival of a normal infant, or may be associated with congenital defects, although there are conflicting reports regarding this in the literature (Packer, 1950; Eichenwald, 1965; Siegel, et al., 1966.).

The Mumps Virus

The mumps virus is also a myxovirus. It varies considerably in shape and size, the diameter ranging from 90 to 340 millimicrons. A shell or nucleocapsid 100 to 150 angstroms deep surrounds an inner helix of nucleoprotein, 9.6 percent of which is ribonucleic acid. The nucleocapsid contains a soluble antigen, while the viral or "V" antigen is found on the surface and on protruding spikes. Both antigens cause hemolysis and hemagglutination and elicit infectivity-neutralizing antibodies, hemagglutination-inhibiting antibodies, and complement fixing antibodies, the latter two of which are commonly used in diagnosis, especially the complement fixation test.

Antibodies may be transferred passively across the placenta to the fetus, are detectable for 40 to 60 days but apparently confer immunity lasting six to nine months. Antibodies have been found in 30 to 50 percent of adults who deny having had mumps. Immunity is quite durable; recurrent attacks occur at a maximum rate of 4 percent. Mumps with or without parotitis confers equal immunity (Horsfall and Tamm, 1965; Horne, et al., 1960).

Pathogenesis and Pathology

The exact pathogenesis is uncertain, but in the usual case the virus may enter the mouth and travel to the salivary gland, usually the parotid, via the salivary duct, and from there to the blood stream, as viremia has been demonstrated early in infection. The mechanism is conjectural for those cases in which distant involvement precedes parotitis. Possibly the virus grows in the respiratory epithelium and then gets into the blood stream. Virus may be recovered from the saliva, mouth washings or cerebrospinal fluid during the first five days of infection in 75 percent of cases and from the urine up to 13 days. The pathogenicity and mortality of mumps seem highest in the youngest patients (Horsfall and Tamm, 1965; Cantell, 1961).

The cytopathic changes caused by mumps virus may be divided into four categories: (1) cytoplasmic inclusion bodies found in cells supporting virus multiplication; (2) cellular damage caused by the cytolytic properties of the virus. Giant-cell formation may also be due to cytolysis; (3) destruction of "hypersensitive" cells caused by a viral antigen devoid of cytolytic activity; and (4) "toxic" lesions induced by the virus in vivo (Cantell, 1961).

The general pathologic changes of mumps are not diagnostic, but they are as follows: (1) Parotid glands: serofibrinous exudate with leukocytes in the connective tissue. The cells of the ducts contain necrotic debris, and polymorphonuclear leukocytes are found in their lumens. (2) Testis: there is considerable destruction of the epithelium of the seminiferous tubules, marked congestion, punctate hemorrhages, and lymphocytic infiltration. In the interstitial tissues edema and serofibrinous exudate occur. (3) Pancreas: again there is congestion, interstitial edema, slight degeneration of the islets of Langerhans and fat necrosis (Horsfall and Tamm). (4) Central nervous system: meningeal thickening with serous exudate, localized fibrinous plaquelike areas and gelatinous edema, the latter surrounding the nerves and basilar areas of the brain, have been reported. (5) There is no clear-cut evidence that mumps in pregnancy has been associated with fetal anomalies.

Clinical Picture of Measles Deafness

Measles is a significant cause of deafness in children. Various series (Bordley and Hardy, 1951; Zonderman, 1959; Shambaugh, et al., 1928; Yearsley, 1934; Kinney, 1953; Lederer, et al., 1926; Goodman, 1949; Simpson 1949.) of deaf children have reported an incidence of measles deafness ranging from 3 to 10 percent. The time of onset of the deafness in measles deafness is unknown. The lesion is a direct involvement of the inner ear probably unrelated to middle-ear or meningeal pathology.

Surveys of deaf patients usually mention measles as a cause of deafness, but the pediatric and otologic literature is surprisingly sparse in describing the clinical aspects of measles deafness except as related to otitis media complicating measles.

Audiometric Findings

Ballantyne (1960) stated that the characteristic audiologic picture is that of a symmetrical, bilateral, partial deafness affecting the high tones more than the low tones and, therefore, giving a gently sloping audiogram, averaging 40 to 50-decibel loss. Experience at the University of Colorado Medical Center has been that the deafness is much more profound. Kinney (1953) reported cases of unilateral deafness with normal hearing in the opposite ear.

Davey (1954) reported vestibular testing in two "postnatal morbilli" patients and reported a unilateral diminished cold caloric in one patient and no response to ice water calorics in either ear of the other patient.

The classic study of Shambaugh Sr., et al. (1928) revealed that 32 of 72 patients with measles inner-ear deafness were totally deaf, 40 partially deaf. Of these 72, 20 had normal vestibular responses, 29 diminished responses, and 23 had no response.

Clinical Picture of Mumps Deafness

Mumps deafness is usually sudden in onset, profound, and may be associated with nausea, vomiting, and vertigo. Tinnitus and a feeling of fullness in the ear may be noted. It is usually unilateral and for this reason may be undiagnosed for years in very young patients. Mumps seems rarely to affect only the vestibular part of the inner ear.

The audiogram usually shows a marked to total neurosensory hearing loss with perhaps some residual hearing below 512 cps. Caloric response may be normal, diminished, or absent.

Pathology

Few published pathological studies of these lesions are available at the present time.

The pathological material available to the authors includes that of 19 ears of 12 patients with probable viral endolabyrinthitis. Two of these are from Dr. Lindsay's laboratory in Chicago, and ten are from Dr. Schuknecht's laboratory in Boston. These cases my be classified as follows:

1. Measles:
   a. a pair of temporal bones showing a subacute bilateral measles endolabyrinthitis;
   b. a pair of ears with a healed bilateral measles lesion.

2. Mumps
   a. a temporal bone showing a healed mumps endolabyrinthitis;
   b. a temporal bone showing a healed endolabyrinthitis, probably either mumps or measles.

3. Five cases of sudden deafness, four unilateral and one bilateral with an interval of 13 years between the onset of deafness in the left and right ears. These are considered to be of probable viral etiology.

4. Three cases of possible viral lesions in severely deafened patients.
   a. an 8-year-old boy who developed a bilateral hearing loss at age two after a severe illness and died of possible measles meningitis;
   b. a 68-year-old deaf-mute who thought that his profound hearing loss was due to whooping cough;
   c. a 25-year-old deaf-mute whose ears showed cochleosaccular degeneration of probable viral origin.

Pathology of Measles Deafness

Moos (1887) described the inner ear changes in a case of deafness following measles. His illustration seems compatible with an early suppurative labyrinthitis complicating either otitis media or meningitis.

Nager (1917) described a case which appears to show a virus lesion complicated by a bacterial labyrinthitis.

Hagens (1937) described temporal bones in a case of measles deafness. Marked widespread destruction of the sensory structures of the inner ear was seen.

Lindsay and Hemenway (1954) reported the findings in a 7-month-old child, (Case 1), who died about three months after the onset of measles of bronchopneumonia and myocardial degeneration.

The inner ear changes were as follows (Figure 1):

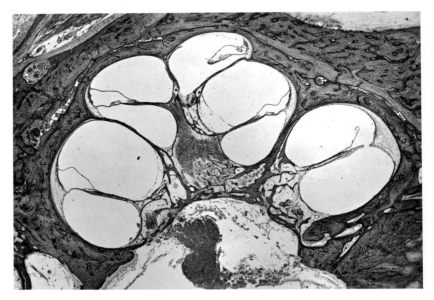

Figure 1, Case 1. Midmodiolar section of the right cochlea showing more marked involvement of the organ of Corti and stria vascularis toward the basal end. The organ of Corti is absent in the basal coil. There is a moderate loss of cochlear neurons in the basal coil.

1. Organ of Corti: There was degeneration. It was absent in the lowest parts of the basal coil. There was corresponding degeneration of the hair cells, pillar cells, and supporting cells.

2. Cochlear neuron: There was moderate loss in the basal coil of each ear.

3. Stria vascularis: There was atrophy, progressively more severe toward the basal end of the cochlea, roughly proportional to the degree of the degeneration of the organ of Corti. In addition, granulomatous lesions containing giant cells were seen in the stria vascularis.

4. Tectorial membrane: Probably the most striking and significant changes were seen in this structure. It was often displaced

medially or laterally from its attachment to the spiral limbus. Often it assumed a rounded shape and was covered by a single layer of flattened cells (Figure 2). In other areas, the tectorial membrane was incorporated into the remnants of the organ of Corti, where it could best be seen using the Mallory stain which colors it blue.

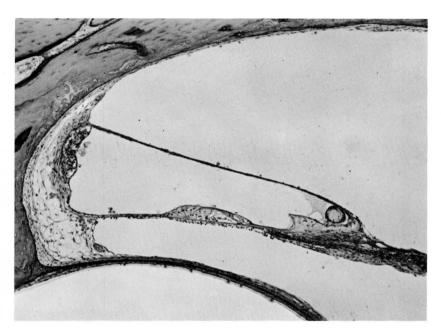

Figure 2, Case 1. The apical coil of the left ear showing hair-cell destruction with the form of the organ of Corti preserved. The tectorial membrane is rounded up, encapsulated, and displaced into the angle between the spiral limbus and Reissner's membrane. The stria vascularis shows a granulomatous lesion.

5. Cochlear duct: Giant cells seemingly liberated from granulomatous lesions were observed floating in the endolymph of the left cochlea (Figure 3).

6. Saccule: In each ear the lateral wall was collapsed, distorted and adherent to a degenerated macula.

7. Utricle: The lumen of the right utricle was filled with pink-staining exudate which was interpreted as serious labyrinthitis (Figure 4).

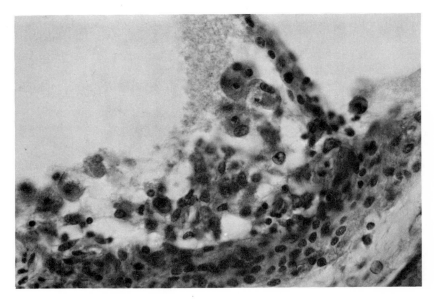

Figure 3, Case 1. Measles granuloma in stria vascularis of apical coil. Granuloma has ruptured and is discharging giant cells into the endolymph.

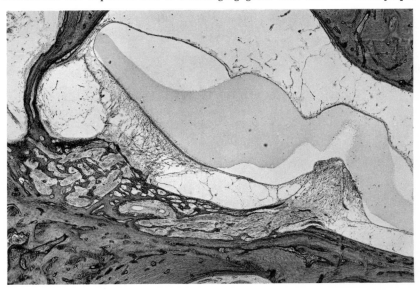

Figure 4, Case 1. Utricle, right ear, showing increased affinity of the endolymph for the stain, indicative of a serous labyrinthitis. There is a lesion within the epithelium of the horizontal canal crista.

The right macula utriculi showed moderate degeneration of the sensory cells, absence of the otolithic membrane and in two areas localized giant cell aggregates reminiscent of measles granulomata (Figure 5). The left utricle was normal.

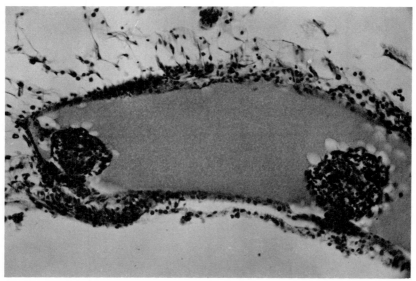

Fig. 5, Case 1. Utricle, right ear, showing two granulomatous lesions consistent with subacute measles.

8. Semicircular canals: The cupulae of all three right semicircular canals were missing. A granulomatous lesion was present in the epithelial layer of the crista of the horizontal semicircular canal of the right ear.

Neither ear showed any evidence of endolymphatic hydrops, nor were any inclusion bodies seen.

This case falls into the category of cochleo-saccular pathology. The various granulomatous changes described above were considered by several pathologists to indicate a subacute measles lesion.

Case 2, Mr. N.A., a 57-year-old man, died of tuberculous meningitis. He had been profoundly deafened since an attack of measles at the age of four. The ears were acquired and processed at Dr. Schuknecht's laboratory in Boston and are previously unreported.

The pathological findings in both ears are similar:

1. (Figure 6) The organ of Corti is either completely absent or severely atrophied.

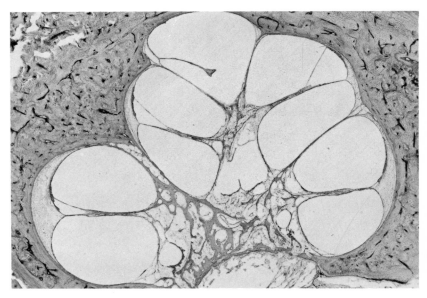

Figure 6, Case 2. Midmodiolar section, right ear, showing almost complete destruction of the organ of Corti with 90 percent loss of cochlear neurons and severe strial atrophy.

2. Cochlear neuron: there is a 90 percent loss of spiral ganglion cells.

3. The saccule shows collapse of the wall, absence of hair cells and irregular masses of tissue in the lumen. (Figure 7)

4. The utricle and all three cristae show degenerative changes. These changes would seem to be the end result of a severe measles endolabyrinthitis.

Pathology of Mumps Deafness

Lindsay, *et al.*, (1960) described a temporal bone of a 6-year-old boy (Case 3) who became totally deaf after an attack of mumps and died of nephritis four years later. The pathology was as follows:

1. Organ of Corti: There was severe degeneration of the organ

of Corti in most of the basal and part of the middle coil with decreasing involvement toward the apical coil. In the apical and upper middle coils hair cells were present in nearly normal numbers.

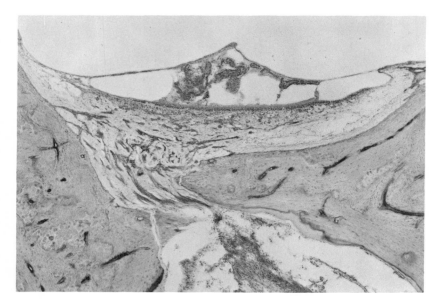

Figure 7, Case 2. The Saccule.

2. Cochlear neuron: Nerve fibers and ganglion cells were some-what decreased in the lower half of the basilar coil (Figure 8).

3. Stria vascularis: There was almost complete absence of the stria vascularis in most of the basal and part of the middle coil with decreasing involvement toward the apical coil. The strial atrophy seemed roughly proportional to that of the organ of Corti at any given level.

4. The tectorial membrane in the basal and part of the middle coil was detached from the limbus spiralis and appeared as a hyaline mass surrounded by a single layer of flattened cells. It lay on the basilar membrane in areas of degenerated or absent organ of Corti. Farther toward the apex it was rolled upon the surface of the limbus near the attachment of Reissner's membrane. In the apical region the tectorial membrane was flattened but still attached (Figure 9).

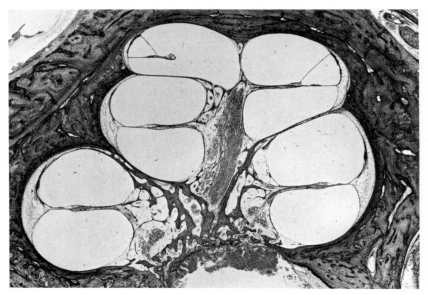

Figure 8, Case 3. Midmodiolar section of the cochlea. There is severe destruction of the organ of Corti, somewhat more marked in the basilar area. This is paralleled by strial atrophy. There is a considerable loss of neurons in the basal coil and marked collapse of Reissner's membrane in the lower-middle and basal coils.

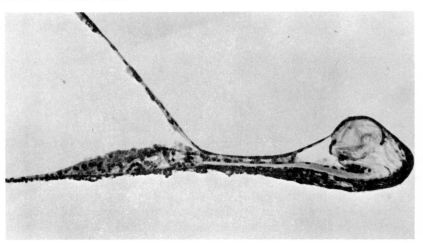

Figure 9, Case 3. Higher power, apical coil shows some degeneration of the organ of Corti but its outline is maintained. The Reissner's membrane is adherent to the remains of the organ of Corti. The tectorial membrane has assumed a rounded shape and is adherent to Reissner's membrane.

5. The vestibular system was essentially normal.

The bone was interpreted as showing a healed lesion. No endolymphatic hydrops was seen in either ear.

Case 4, Mr. R.P., which is from Dr. Schuknecht's laboratory, is being presented as a case of viral endolabyrinthitis. This 40-year-old man died of a pulmonary embolus. He had had a severely deafened left ear since boyhood. Further historical data is lacking. The pathology is as follows:

1. The organ of Corti is severely atrophied throughout (Figure 10a).

2. There is a severe loss of cochlear neurons with only a few remaining in the apical region.

3. In some regions the tectorial membrane is balled up, lying on the limbus and encapsulated in a single layer of flattened cells (Figure 10b).

4. The saccular epithelium is degenerated with an almost total loss of hair cells. The otolithic membrane is atrophied.

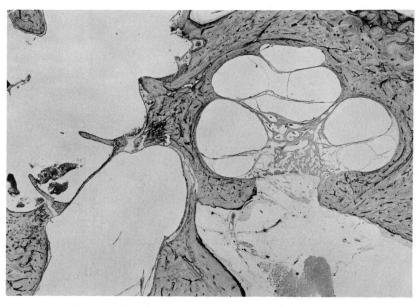

Figure 10a, Case 4. There is a severe atrophy of the organ of Corti accompanied by severe loss of cochlear neurons. The cochlea and saccule show a severe hydrops, the cause of which is unexplained.

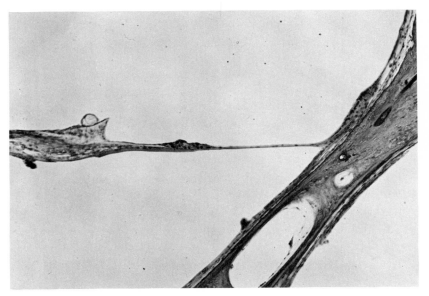

Figure 10b, Case 4. High-power middle coil. The organ of Corti is represented by a small irregular mound of undifferentiated cells. The tectorial membrane is rolled up and is lying on top of the remains of the spiral limbus.

5. There is a severe unexplained hydrops of both the auditory and vestibular labyrinth.

Impression: The pathology in this ear is cochleo-saccular and is probably of viral origin. The findings are compatible with either mumps or measles.

The Pathology of Sudden Deafness

Schuknecht, *et al.* (1962) described the pathology in the temporal bones of four patients who had sudden unilateral deafness. The following is a resumé of these four cases plus an additional case.

Case 5, Mrs. A.P., had the onset of profound deafness in the right ear following a head cold at the age of 39 and died 20 years later of adenocarcinoma of the colon. Audiometry three weeks before death revealed a recruiting right sensorineural hearing loss which ranged from 40 decibels in the low frequencies to 70 decibels in the high frequencies. Histologic examination of the right temporal bone revealed the following:

1. Organ of Corti was shrunken with moderate hair cell loss except in the basal 5 mm where there was a total loss of hair cells.

2. The tectorial membrane was shrunken.

3. The macula sacculi was devoid of hair cells, but supporting cells were present. The saccular wall was ruptured, collapsed and adherent to the underlying shrunken otolithic membrane. (Figure 11)

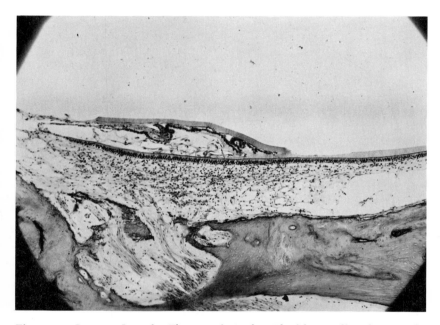

Figure 11, Case 5. Saccule. The macula is devoid of hair cells. The saccular wall is ruptured, collapsed, and adherent to the underlying shrunken otolithic membrane.

4. The utricle was normal.

5. The semicircular canals were normal.

The picture, then, was of cochleosaccular degeneration almost certainly due to a virus infection. The left temporal bone was normal.

The second ear, Case 6, Mr. H.H., was obtained by Dr. Beekhuis and sent to Dr. Schuknecht's laboratory. The patient was a

59-year-old male who had the onset of sudden severe right-sided deafness three days after having a head cold. Audiometry done shortly after showed a profound sensorineural loss. He died nine days after of a coronary occlusion. Histologic examination of the right temporal bone revealed the following:

1. Organ of Corti: There was considerable shrinkage of the organ of Corti in 10 to 16 mm region.

2. Stria vascularis: there was atrophy of the stria vascularis throughout the basal 16 mm of the cochlea.

3. Tectorial membrane: the tectorial membrane was atrophied throughout the basal 16 mm of the cochlea. In some areas the tectorial membrane appeared as a homogeneous sphere encased in flattened cells and lying on the limbus. In the apical region the tectorial membrane was missing entirely.

4. The vestibular organs appeared within normal limits.

Impression: Probable viral endolabyrinthitis.

Case 7, Mr. P.C., a 63-year-old man who experienced a sudden attack of vertigo, nausea and vomiting, accompanied by a loss of hearing in his left ear. The vertigo soon subsided, but a profound left-sided hearing loss persisted. Six weeks later he was found to have a diminished caloric response on the affected side. There was no measurable hearing in this ear. He died four years later of Laennec's cirrhosis and cardiac disease. The pathology of the left temporal bone is as follows:

1. The organ of Corti is missing on the basal 17.5 mm of the cochlea. In the remainder of the cochlea supporting cells are present without hair cells. (Figures 12a and 12b)

2. Cochlear neuron: There is a 50 percent loss of ganglion cells in the lower basal turn. The number of ganglion cells gradually increases to normal at 23 mm. (Figure 12c)

3. The stria vascularis is mildly atrophic or possibly within normal limits.

4. The tectorial membrane, spiral ligament, and Reissner's membrane appear normal.

5. Saccule, utricle, and canals: The cristae and maculae appear normal; thus no pathological explanation of the diminished caloric response can be given.

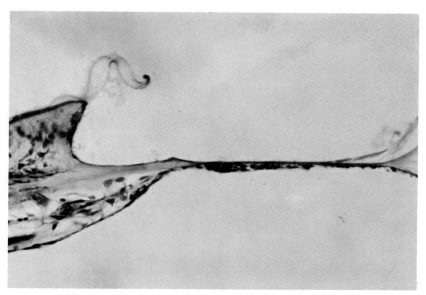

Figure 12a, Case 7. High-power basal turn. The organ of Corti is absent. The cochlear neuron fibers are missing. The tectorial membrane is normal.

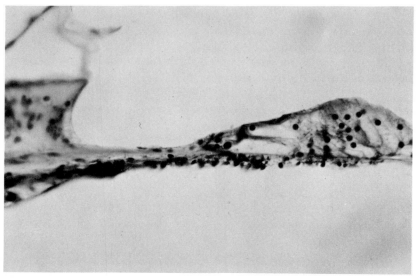

Figure 12b, Case 7. Organ of Corti middle coil. There is preservation of the supporting cells. No hair cells are seen.

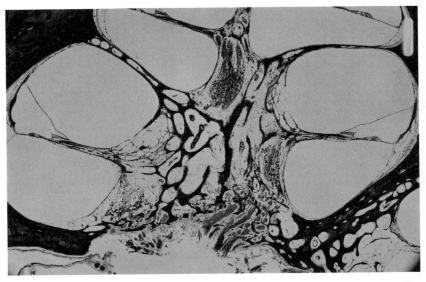

Figure 12c, Case 7. Midmodiolar section shows loss of ganglion cells in the basal turn. There is a suggestion of mild strial atrophy. The tectorial membrane is normal.

Impression: Probable viral endolabyrinthitis.

The temporal bones of Case 8, Mrs. B.W., were prepared in Dr. Ruedi's laboratory in Zurich. They were examined in Dr. Schuknecht's temporal-bone laboratory. The patient apparently had good hearing in early life but suddenly lost the hearing in her left ear at the age of 52. Thirteen years later she suddenly developed total deafness in the right ear. She died at age 85 from bronchopneumonia after a fractured femur.

Pathology—Left ear (Figure 13):

1. The organ of Corti is entirely missing in the basal half of the cochlea. A few hair cells remain in the apex.

2. Cochlear neuron: There is a severe loss of cochlear neurons varying from 90 percent at the basal end to 30 to 60 percent at the apical end.

3. In addition, there is severe atrophy of the stria vascularis with only isolated areas remaining in the apical half of the cochlea.

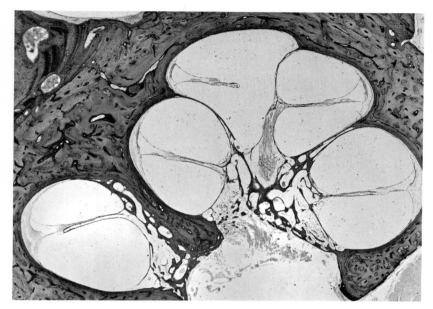

Figure 13, Case 8. Midmodiolar section organ of Corti, left ear. There is severe atrophy of the organ of Corti accompanied by corresponding loss of cochlear neurons and atrophy of the stria vascularis.

4. The vestibular organs are normal.

Pathology—Right ear:

1. Organ of Corti: There is a loss of about 75 percent of the hair cells throughout the cochlea.

2. Cochlear neuron: About 60 percent of the cochlear neurons are absent in the basal 10 mm.

3. Stria vascularis: There is a 1 mm segment of atrophy of the stria vascularis at the 20 mm region.

4. The vestibular organs are normal.

Impression: Probable viral endolabyrinthitis, bilateral.

Case 9, Mrs. B.H., was a 44-year-old woman who suddenly developed a left sensorineural hearing loss with incomplete loudness recruitment. Caloric tests were normal. Four months later an audiogram showed a 30-decibel sensorineural hearing loss for frequencies up to 1,000 cps and a profound loss for higher frequencies. She died eleven months later.

The pathology was as follows (Figure 14):

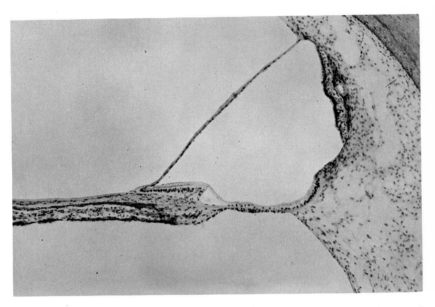

Figure 14, Case 9. Basal turn: Organ of Corti is replaced by a layer of flattened cells. The tectorial membrane is atrophic and adherent to the remains of the organ of Corti. There is some strial atrophy, similar to that present on the other ear and therefore not considered to the associated with the virus lesion.

1. The organ of Corti is flattened and the hair cells are missing in the basal 11 mm of the cochlea. The organ of Corti lesion is considered responsible for the severe high-frequency loss.

2. Cochlear neuron population is normal.

3. There is atrophy of the stria vascularis in the middle and apical turns. The strial atrophy is similar to that seen in the opposite ear and is thought to account for the 30-decibel loss.

4. The vestibular organs are normal.

This is considered to be a probable virus lesion.

Three additional cases from Dr. Schuknecht's laboratory that may be of viral etiology are presented. All had severe, bilateral hearing loss and two were considered to be deaf-mutes.

Case 10, R.O., was an 8-year-old boy whose temporal bones were obtained by Dr. Charles Kinney. The patient apparently developed normally until the age of two when he suffered from a severe illness which was probably a form of encephalitis. He developed a spastic condition and had considerable residual hearing, but his hearing was considered to be fairly good. He progressed satisfactorily in a school for the deaf until he developed fatal measles encephalitis.

The pathological findings are as follows (Figure 15):

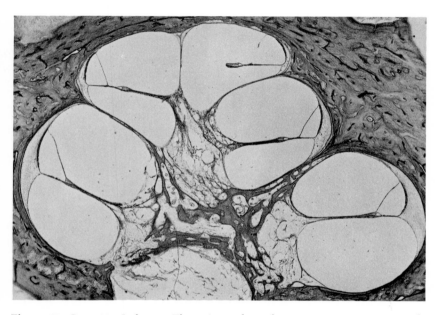

Figure 15, Case 10. Left ear. There is moderately severe postmortem autolysis, The striking feature is complete absence of the cochlear neurons. Efferent fibers persist and are best seen going to the apical region.

Right ear: Moderately severe autolysis makes interpretation of the sensory structures very difficult. The striking finding is the total absence of cochlear nerve fibers and ganglion cells. The efferent fibers persist and are visible, especially to the apical turn.

The superior division of the vestibular nerve shows a moderately severe loss of nerve fibers.

Left ear: The findings are similar to the right except the superior division of the vestibular nerve is normal.

Summary: This is a complicated case. Two separate infections are recorded in the history, and postmortem autolysis makes interpretation difficult. It is quite possible, however, that he suffered a partial hearing loss due to a virus infection when two years of age, and that the remainder of the damage was done by his terminal attack of measles.

Case 11, Mr. E.M., was a 68-year-old deaf-mute. He indicated that he had been unable to hear since an attack of whooping cough at the age of eight months.

The pathology in both ears is as follows:

1. There are advanced changes in the organ of Corti. It is absent throughout the lower half of the cochlea. There is severe degeneration of the organ of Corti in the apical half of the cochlea with complete absence of hair cells (Figure 16).

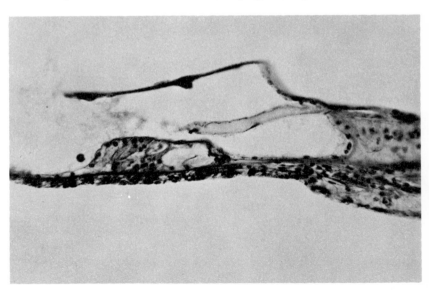

Figure 16, Case 11. High power of the organ of Corti in the upper middle coil. There is a complete absence of hair cells but the supporting cells of the organ of Corti remain intact. The tectorial membrane is normal.

2. Cochlear neuron: In the lower half of the cochlea there is almost total loss of cochlear neurons.

3. Stria vascularis: There is moderately severe atrophy of the stria vascularis in the apical turn.

4. The tectorial membrane and Reissner's membrane appear normal.

5. The vestibular organs are normal.

Impression: These ears show severe bilateral destruction of the organ of Corti with secondary nerve degeneration consistent with a diagnosis of viral endolabyrinthitis. Against this interpretation is the history of onset during whooping cough which is generally considered as a cause of deafness in childhood. Pertussis is a much less frequent cause of deafness than viral disease, and no pathological findings in the former have been recorded. Moreover, deaf-mutes frequently give inaccurate information as to the cause of their handicap. Therefore the authors consider a viral etiology to be more probable.

Case 12, Mr. A.L., is an ear that Dr. Schuknecht obtained from Dr. Ruedi's laboratory. The patient was a 25-year-old deaf-mute about whom little was known. His case is included in this report because the findings are consistent with a viral endolabyrinthitis. Historical data is not available which would differentiate a congenital virus lesion, rubella, from an acquired lesion.

1. Organ of Corti: There is severe degeneration of the organ of Corti with very few hair cells remaining.

2. Cochlear neuron: Fifty percent of the ganglion cells are missing.

3. Stria vascularis: severe diffuse strial atrophy is seen.

4. The tectorial membrane assumes a rounded shape and is displaced medially.

5. The saccular wall is collapsed and adherent to the macular area which shows marked hair-cell loss.

Discussion

At the present time there are no pathological changes which are specifically diagnostic of acquired viral endolabyrinthitis. As more pathological material accumulates, however, a series of changes emerges that appears to differ qualitatively and quantitatively from other lesions which might present a similar picture. The history, if available, is of vital importance in differentiating congenital lesions such as rubella and hereditary deafness from acquired viral disease. The history of onset during a known or suspected viral infection is very valuable. Development of the deafness in infancy or childhood makes a viral etiology more likely. Results of audiometric and caloric tests are of somewhat less value in reaching a pathologic diagnosis.

One of the main problems is to assess the etiology of sudden deafness which occurs in adults. The two most commonly considered causes of sudden deafness are a viral endolabyrinthitis and a vascular occlusion due to a thrombus or an embolus. There may well be other causes. The pathological material presented here consists of six ears which clinically were diagnosed as sudden deafness. All of these have been interpreted as viral lesions. A paradoxical situation exists in our knowledge of viral lesions and vascular obstruction. All of the available material on viral lesions is on human material, whereas all information on vascular obstruction has been acquired from animal experiments (Perlman et al., 1965; Kimura and Perlman, 1956, 1958). Efforts are currently underway to produce experimental viral endolabyrinthitis. If these experiments are successful our knowledge of these diseases will increase considerably.

The chart (opposite) summarizes the pathological findings in viral endolabyrinthitis, in experimental vascular occlusion, and in hereditary deafness of the Scheibe type (Ormerod, 1960; Schuknecht, et al., 1965).

It is the impression of the essayists that after examining a series of temporal bones suspected of showing virus lesions certain patterns begin to develop. While there are no findings pathognomonic of viral disease in the inner ear, the lesion can usually be diagnosed in a given case.

COCHLEA

	DISTRIBUTION OF PATHOLOGIC CHANGE	ORGAN OF CORTI	COCHLEAR NEURON	STRIA VASCULARIS
Viral Lesions (all human ears)	Nearly always more marked toward basal end.	Always involved in these specimens. Degree of destruction varies from hair-cell loss only to complete absence, more marked toward basal end.	Usually involved but not always. Destruction usually is proportional to the degree of destruction of the supporting cells of the organ of Corti.	Usually involved. Amount of atrophy varies in different regions—may be restricted to one area. Often more pronounced toward basal end.
Vascular Obstruction (all animal experiments)	Diffuse involvement	Widespread degeneration throughout the entire cochlea no predilection for basal end.	Severe, diffuse degeneration. More marked than organ of Corti.	Widespread degeneration throughout.
Hereditary Deafness— Scheibe Type (both humans and animals)	Diffuse involvement	Constantly involved throughout the entire extent. May be seen as a mound of undifferentiated cells resembling fetal epithelium.	Normal	Striking changes are seen which may be diagnostic. The stria is avascular, compressed, and shows irregular folds and projections into the cochlear duct. Changes may vary according to the species of animal.

COCHLEA

	TECTORIAL MEMBRANE	SPIRAL LIGAMENT	COCHLEAR DUCT
Viral Lesions (all human ears)	Often involved. A frequent observation is that it assumes a circular shape surrounded by flattened cells and is displaced medially or laterally. May be incorporated into remains of organ of Corti. May be normal or atrophic.	Normal	Usually normal. May be collapsed. One case showed a hydrops.
Vascular Obstruction (all animal experiments)	Normal	Loss of cellularity near the attachment of the basal membrane.	Eventually invaded by fibrous tissue and bone. (endo-labyrinthitis ossificans)
Hereditary Deafness— Scheibe Type (both humans and animals)	Diffusely distorted and flattened. Occasionally it may assume a round, encapsulated form.	Normal	Some species (Dalmatian dog) show uniform collapse. Reissner's membrane is adherent to the remnants of the organ of Corti and stria vascularis. Other species show normal duct.

VESTIBULAR ORGANS

	SACCULE	UTRICLE	CANALS
Viral Lesions (all human ears)	Abnormal in 6 out of 15 ears in which information is available. Usually shows severe distortion of the lateral wall with adhesions to the macular area. Sometimes amorphous tissue develops in the lumen. The sensory cells show severe loss and the supporting cells are often degenerated. Occasionally only the hair cells are missing.	Occasional involvement	Occasional involvement
Vascular Obstruction (all animal experiments)	Degenerated.	Degenerated	Degenerated
Hereditary Deafness— Scheibe Type (both humans and animals)	Saccular wall is distorted, collapsed, and adherent to the macula which contains fetal-type epithelium.	Normal	Degenerated

Summary and Conclusions

1. Seventeen temporal bones from 11 patients have been presented as representing known or suspected acquired viral lesions of the inner ear. Another case is briefly described which reveals a lesion almost certainly of viral etiology, but the history is not available which would differentiate a congenital (rubella) from an acquired disease.

2. One pair of ears reveals a subacute viral lesion (measles). The remaining ears show the residual destruction in the ear from previous virus infections.

3. The route of infection is not clear at this time, but it is probably the bloodstream.

4. A chart has been developed comparing the findings in viral lesions, vascular obstruction, and hereditary deafness. The authors conclude that while there are no pathognomic changes in the viral ears, qualitative and quantitative analysis of the pathology will usually lead to a diagnosis.

5. The importance of the history and clinical findings is stressed.

6. The need for experimental observations on viral lesions is evident.

7. Many more well documented human ears will have to be examined before this lesion is truly understood. With the impetus given to temporal-bone pathology by the temporal-bone banks program of the Deafness Research Foundation, the authors are confident that the necessary material will soon be forthcoming.

References

Ballantyne, J. C. 1960. *Deafness.* Boston: Little, Brown, & Co.

Bordley, J. E., and W. G. Hardy. 1951. "The Etiology of Deafness in Young Children." *Acta oto-laryng.,* **40**:72–79.

Cantell, K. 1961. "Mumps Virus." *Advances Virus Res.,* **8**:123–164.

Davey, P. R. 1954. "Observations on Equilibrium in Deaf Children." *J. Laryng. & Otol.,* **68**:329–330.

Dyer, I. 1940. "Measles Complicating Pregnancy: Report of 24 Cases With Three Instances of Congenital Measles." *South. M. J.,* **33**:601–604.

Eichenwald, H. F. 1965. "The Placental 'Barrier' and Infections of the Fetus." *Birth Defects*, **1**(April):74–75.

Goodman, A. 1949. "Residual Capacity to Hear of Pupils in Schools for the Deaf." *J. Laryng. & Otol.*, **63**:551, 551–579, 1949.

Habel, K., and J. P. Utz. 1960. "Mumps." *Pediat. Clin. N. Am.*, **7**:979–988.

Horne, R. W., A. P. Waterson, P. Wildy, and A. E. Farnham. 1960. "The Structure and Composition of Myxoviruses. I. Electron Microscope Studies of the Structure of Myxovirus Particles by Negative Staining Techniques." *Virology*, **11**:79–98.

Horsfall, F. L., Jr., and I. Tamm. 1965. *Viral and Rickettsial Infections of Man*, ed. 4. Philadelphia: J. B. Lippincott, Co.

Kempe, C. H. and V. A. Fulginiti. 1965. "The Pathogenesis of Measles Virus Infection." *Arch. fur die Gesamte Virusforschung*, XVI (Heft 1–5), 103–128.

Kimura, R. and H. B. Perlman. 1956. "Extensive Venous Obstruction of the Labyrinth." *Ann. Otol. Rhin. & Laryng.*, **65**:332–350.

Kimura, R., and H. B. Perlman. 1958. "Arterial Obstruction of the Labyranth; Part 1. Cochlear Changes." *Ann. Otol. Rhin. & Laryng.*, **67**:5–40.

Kinney, C. E. 1953. "Hearing Impairment in Children." *Laryngoscope*, **63**:220–226.

Lederer, L., A. Denker, and O. Kahler. 1926. Handbuch der Hals Nasen Ohren Heilkunde. **2**:333. Ed. by Alfred Denker and Otto Kahler. Berlin: Springer.

Lewy, A., and E. Hagens. 1937. "Report of the Chicago Committee on Otitic Meningitis." *Laryngoscope*, **47**:761–775.

Lindsay, J. R. 1959. "Sudden Deafness Due to Virus Infection." *Arch. Otol.*, **69**:13–18.

Lindsay, J. R., P. R. Davey, and P. H. Ward. 1960. "Inner Ear Pathology In Deafness Due to Mumps." *Ann. Otol. Rhin. & Laryng.*, **69**:918–935.

Lindsay, J. R., and W. G. Hemenway. 1954. "Inner Ear Pathology Due to Measles." *Ann. Otol. Rhin. & Laryng.*, **63**:754–771.

Lindsay, J. R., and J. J. Zuidema. 1950. "Inner Ear Deafness of Sudden Onset." *Laryngoscope*, **60**:238–263.

Moos, von S. 1887. "Untersuchungen über Pilzinvasion des Labyrinthes im Gefolge von Masern." *Ztschr. Ohrenh.*, **18**:97–154.

Nager, von F. R. 1907. "Beitrage zur Histologie der erworkenen, Taubstummheit." *Ztschr. Ohrenh.*, **54**:217.

Ormerod, F. C. 1960. "The Pathology of Congenital Deafness." *J. Laryng. & Otol.*, **74**:919–948.

Packer, A. D. 1950. "The Influence of Maternal Measles (Morbilli) on the Newborn Child." *M. J. Australia,* **1**:835–837.

Perlman, H. B., R. Kimura, and C. Fernandez. 1959. "Experiments on Temporary Obstruction of the Internal Auditory Artery." *Laryngoscope,* **69**:591–613.

Saunders, W. H., and W. H. Lippy. 1959. "Sudden Deafness and Bell's Palsy: A Common Cause." *Ann. Otol. Rhin. & Laryng.,* **68**:830–837.

Schuknecht, H. F., J. Benitez, J. Beekhuis, M. Igarashi, G. Singleton, and L. Ruedi. 1962. "The Pathology of Sudden Deafness." *Laryngoscope,* **72**:1142–1157.

Schuknecht, H. F., M. Igarashi, and R. Gacek. 1965. "The Pathological Types of Cochleo-Saccular Degeneration." *Acta oto-laryng.,* **59**: 154–167.

Shambaugh, G. E., E. W. Hagen, J. W. Holderman, and R. W. Watkins. 1928. "Statistical Studies of the Children in the Public Schools for the Deaf." *Arch. Otol.,* **7**:424–513.

Siegel, M., H. T. Fuerst, and N. S. Peress. 1966. "Comparative Fetal Mortality in Maternal Virus Diseases: A Prospective Study on Rubella, Measles, Mumps, Chickenpox, and Hepatitis." *New England J. Med.,* **274**:768–771.

Simpson, R. R. 1949. "The Causes of Perceptive Deafness." *Proc. Roy. Soc. Med.,* **42**:536–540.

Ward, P. H., J. R. Lindsay, and N. E. Warner. 1965. "Cytomegalic Inclusion Disease Affecting the Temporal Bone." *Laryngoscope,* **75**:628–636.

Waterson, A. P., J. G. Cruickshank, G. D. Laurence, and A. D. Kanarek. 1961. "The Nature of Measles Virus." *Virology,* **15**:379–382.

Whetnall, E., and D. B. Fry. 1964. *The Deaf Child.* London: The Whitefriars Press., Ltd.

Yearsley, M. 1934. "An Analysis of Over 4000 Cases of Educational Deafness Studied During the Past 25 Years." *Brit. J. Child Dis.,* **31**: 177–192, **31**:277–290.

Zonderman, B. 1959. "The Pre-School Nerve-Deaf Child: Study of Etiologic Factors." *Laryngoscope,* **69**:54–89.

CHAPTER **9**   JOHN E. BORDLEY,
PATRICK E. BROOKHOUSER,
JANET HARDY, AND WILLIAM G. HARDY

OBSERVATIONS ON THE EFFECT OF PRENATAL RUBELLA IN HEARING
A Preliminary Report on the Baltimore Epidemic of 1963-1965

MODERN interest in prenatal rubella as a cause of congenital defects began with the Australian epidemic of 1939–1941. After this epidemic Gregg (1941) described congenital cataracts in babies of mothers who had rubella during the first three months of pregnancy. Swan (1944) was the first to describe deaf-mutism in these rubella babies. Other anomalies that have become associated with this infection are patent ducts arteriosus and other cardiovascular defects, microcephaly, general stunting of growth, and mental retardation.

Carruthers (1945) reported that in 147 births following prenatal rubella which resulted in injured infants, 116 children showed severe deafness.

Goodhill (1950), working from a questionnaire sent to mothers of 904 profoundly deafened children, concluded that maternal rubella was the "potential cause" of deafness in 25 percent of the cases.

Jackson and Fisch (1958) reviewed 57 children, aged 3 to 5 years, who gave histories of maternal rubella during the first 18 weeks of pregnancy. Fourteen suffered from hearing impairment.

This study was supported in part by the National Institutes of Health Grant Number ND 02371, and in part by the Subcommittee for Hearing in Children of the Conservation of Hearing Committee of the A.A.O.O.

123

Barr and Lundstrom (1961) in Stockholm studied 752 children with severe hearing impairments. They found that all cases of congenital rubella deafness stemmed from maternal rubella in the first four months of pregnancy. In a prospective phase of this study, they examined 44 out of 46 children who had a maternal history of rubella during the first five months of pregnancy. The incidence of hearing loss among these children was 22 percent for cases of rubella within the first 4 months of pregnancy, the loss was found to be severe in 8 percent of the patients tested. No deafness was found for rubella of later onset. Audiograms of the rubella-deafened children had a typical asymmetrical appearance, the graphs being flat and the loss sometimes unilateral. Vestibular functions were normal.

Carruthers (1945) made the first report of histological changes occurring in the inner ear following prenatal rubella. Tondurry (1951), Schall, et al. (1951) Kamerbeek (1949), Nager (1952), and Lindsay, et al. (1953) have since reported studies on temporal bones received from children of women suffering from rubella during their pregnancies. The pathological changes noted in the affected ears have been seen around the cochlear duct and the saccule.

To date there have been no correlations between virological studies and the morbidity of the disease as it relates to hearing. The present report has tried to bring together some of the laboratory findings and relate them to clinical and pathological studies of a group of children born following maternal infection by rubella at the time of pregnancy.

An epidemic of rubella occurred in the eastern states in the spring of 1963, peaked in March and April 1964, and subsided finally in the spring of 1965. It has provided an unequalled opportunity to make observations in depth on the effect of maternal rubella during pregnancy on fetal outcome. The isolation of the rubella virus by Parkman, Beischer, and Artenstein (1962), and Weller and Neva (1962) made definitive diagnostic study possible. During the Baltimore epidemic these techniques could be applied to study virologically- and/or serologically-confirmed cases, in relation to eventual pathology.

The studies on this epidemic have been carried out at the Johns Hopkins Hospital by Dr. John Sever, the Perinatal Infectious Diseases Laboratory, NINDB, and members of various interested groups within the Medical Institutions. These studies have been co-ordinated through the facilities of the Johns Hopkins Collaborative Project on Cerebral Palsy under the direction of Dr. Janet Hardy. The first reports were published in February 1966. (Monif, et al., 1966; Hardy, et al., 1964, 1965, 1966; Alford, et al., 1964; Sever, et al., 1964; Sever, et al., 1965)

Today a preliminary report will be made on a selected group of children in the rubella study. Time permits the recitation of only a few observations made on this group and the presentation of selected sections from a pair of temporal bones obtained from a child who was studied in this group.

TABLE I

TOTAL CASES IN STUDY	79
(A) CASES WITH POSITIVE VIRUS	47
(B) CASES WITH POSITIVE SEROLOGY	32

The study group consists of the first 79 children (Table I) whose prenatal exposure to rubella has been confirmed by (1) positive viral cultures from the throat, urine, organs of the child, or the placenta, or (2) positive serological reactions demonstrated on the blood of the child and/or its mother. Many children with the stigma of prenatal rubella are not included in this study. It is expected that approximately 300 children will eventually be in the study. Among them will be some 100 whose disease has been confirmed by the above criteria.

In the study group, 47 children exhibited positive virus cultures. In many cases the virus survived a surprisingly long time, positive cultures being obtained at 4 and 6 months post-delivery in a number of instances, and one child had a positive culture at 15 months (Table II). One child whose mother had had rubella

TABLE II

CLINICAL CASES OF RUBELLA

	Virus Pos.	Serology Pos.
PRECONCEPTION	1	1
1st TRIMESTER	21	6
2nd TRIMESTER	3	11
3rd TRIMESTER	1	1
TOTAL	26	19

two months before conception exhibited live virus at birth. He suffered from cardiac anomalies and died before his hearing was tested. The child of a second preconception rubella showed a positive serological reaction and cardiac defect. Positive cultures were obtained from the placenta in 5 instances when there was no positive culture from the child. Fifteen children exhibited positive virus cultures where there was no history of prenatal rubella or maternal exposure to rubella. Ten positive sero-

TABLE III

SUBCLINICAL CASES OF RUBELLA

	Virus Pos.	Serology Pos.
HISTORY OF EXPOSURE		
1st TRIMESTER	5	
2nd TRIMESTER		1
3rd TRIMESTER	1	2
NO POSITIVE HISTORY	15	10
TOTAL	21	13

logical reactions (Table III) were obtained in women giving no history of prenatal rubella or exposure to rubella. Their children bear the stigma of prenatal rubella.

In the group of 79 children, 34 mothers suffered from subclinical rubella which could be identified only by cultures or serum studies. Eight of these mothers gave a history of exposure during pregnancy.

To date, 49 children have completed hearing screening tests, based on the Ewing test techniques, and follow-up retests, employing the Ewing techniques and hearing evaluations employing a special speech hearing evaluator, with a frequency range between 50 and 10,000 c.p.s. This evaluator employs human voice, white noise, high-pitched rattles, and squeeky toys. A passing mark requires consistent responses, preferably including localization at ranges of 30 decibels s.p.l. Failures are recorded when there are no consistent responses to sound at or above 50 decibels s.p.l. Inconclusive tests are to be followed by electroencephalographic tests and electrodermal studies.

Thirty-one of the 49 children tested to date failed their screening tests, which were carried out in the Perinatal Center by technicians trained in the Hearing and Speech Center. Retests were done on all 49 children in the Hearing and Speech Center, under the direct supervision of members of the senior staff.

TABLE IV

HEARING RETEST RESULTS (49 CASES)

	No.	Passed	Incon.	Failed
VIRUS-POSITIVE	26	(10) 38.5%	0	(16) 61.5%
SEROPOSITIVE	23	(13) 56.5%	(2) 8.7%	(8) 34.8%
TOTAL	49	(23) 47.0%	(2) 4.0%	(24) 49.0%

Twenty-six children in the virus-positive group were retested (Table IV). Ten (38.5 percent) passed the retest, while 16 (61.5 percent) failed. Twenty-three of the seropositive group were re-tested. Thirteen (56.5 percent) passed, 2 (8.7 percent) gave questionable responses, and 8 (34.8 percent) failed to meet criteria. The total group of 49 showed failures in 49 percent, satisfactory hearing in 47 percent, and questionable hearing in 4 percent.

TABLE V

AGE OF DETERMINATION OF ABNORMAL HEARING

Age	Percent
WITHIN 6 MONTHS	20.8
WITHIN 12 MONTHS	66.7
WITHIN 18 MONTHS	87.5
WITHIN 24 MONTHS	95.8

The test-retest (Table V) procedures were completed in 20.8 percent of the group within the first six months postpartum, 66.7 percent were completed within the first year, 87.5 percent within the first 18 months and 95.8 percent within the first 24 months.

A review of the most frequent defects found in the 49 hearing-tested children shows (Table VI) that the greatest injury has been suffered by those children from whom live virus could be cultured after birth. The children least affected in the virus positive group were those where positive cultures were obtained only from the mother's placenta. In the virus positive group, the children failing their hearing test-retest (Table VII) showed the greatest number of associated defects.

TABLE VI

CORRELATION OF DEFECTS
GROUP I—VIRUS-POSTIVE / HEARING NORMAL

Case #	Premie	Ocular	Cardiac	Retarded	Microcephaly	Placenta
1	X	X	X	X		
3	X		X	X		
28	X		X			
30			X			
31				X	X	
32			X			X
34						X
37						X
42						X
47				X		

TABLE VII

CORRELATION OF DEFECTS
GROUP II—VIRUS-POSITIVE / HEARING ABNORMAL

Case #	Premie	Ocular	Cardiac	Retarded	Microcephaly
2	X	X	X	X	X
6	X	X	X	X	X
7	X		X	X	X
8	X	X	X	X	
9	X	X	X	X	X
11	X	X	X	X	X
24	X	X	X		
4		X	X		
12		X	X		
13		X		X	
14		X	X	X	
15		X	X	X	X
16		X	X	X	
21		X	X	X	X
22				X	·X
27		X	X		X

Among the serological positives (Table VIII) the associated defects were about the same for all children, regardless of passing or failing the hearing test-retest (Table IX). As a group, these

TABLE VIII

CORRELATION OF DEFECTS
GROUP III—SEROLOGY POSITIVE / HEARING NORMAL

Case #	Premie	Ocular	Cardiac	Retarded	Microcephaly
48	X		X	X	
51	X		X		X
54	X			X	X
58	X			X	
49				X	X
55					
56					
59					
60				X	
62					
63				X	
78					
61					

TABLE IX

CORRELATION OF DEFECTS
GROUP IV—SEROLOGY POSITIVE / HEARING ABNORMAL

Case #	Premie	Ocular	Cardiac	Retarded	Microcephaly
64				X	X
77		X		X	
80				X	X
50				X	
53				X	
66			X	X	
68			X	X	
70				X	X
75					
76				X	

children were much less damaged than the virus-positive children. The defects occurring most frequently in the 49 hearing-tested children were prematurity, occular changes, cardiac maldevelopment, peripheral pulmonary stenosis, retarded development, microcephaly, and hearing loss. There was a close relationship between the occurrence of hearing test failures, occular changes, and cardiac maldevelopment in the virus-positive children.

While the majority of positive viral isolations resulted when rubella had occurred during the first trimester, rubella virus was recovered from the throat of a child whose mother had rubella at 17 weeks' gestation. Children born following prenatal rubella in the first trimester showed the highest hearing test-retest failure. An especially disturbing finding, however, is that 23 percent of the children born following infection during the second trimester failed their hearing tests.

Two temporal bones have been processed to date. They were obtained from a virus positive boy, age 31 days. He had failed to show any response to simple sound stimuli, but no assessment could be made of his hearing. His autopsy revealed many defects and virus could be cultured from nearly all of the organs, including the eyes. At the time of death the carotid arteries were perfused with 5 percent formalin, and the autopsy was done two hours after death. The processing of the sections was completed April 21, 1966.

Both ears show Scheibe-type changes in the scala media and the saccule. The right ear appears to have sustained more injury than the left.

The cochlea of the right ear (Figure 1) shows a collapsed Reissner's membrane which appears to have become adherent to the stria vascularis (Figure 2) and plastered against the organ of Corti. The stria itself is small and appears to lack the normal number of capillaries. The tectorial membrane is compressed into the internal sulcus and is covered in some areas by a single-layered membrane, extending under Reissner's membrane. The hair cells are present, and no change could be seen in the pillar cells. The osseous spiral lamina is well filled with nerve fibers, and the spiral ganglion cells appear plentiful. In several areas, the internal sulcus is filled with a pink staining material. The external sulcus, basilar membrane, and vas prominens are normal. The apical turn (Figure 3) shows less displacement of Reissner's

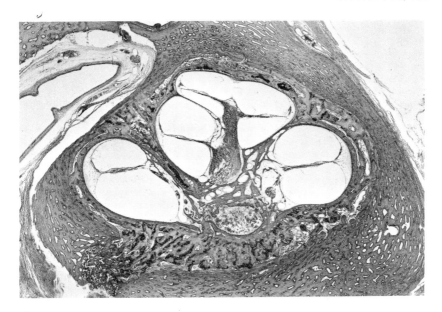

Figure 1

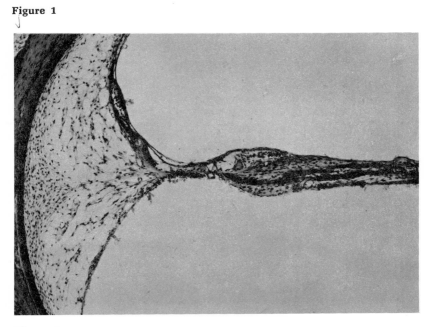

Figure 2

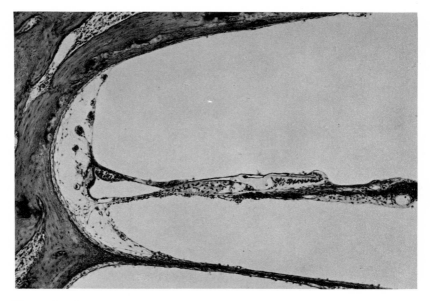

Figure 3

membrane than do the middle and basal turns. The spiral ligament is normal.

The saccule is partially collapsed (Figure 4). The thin portion
of the membrane appears to be adherent at one point to the
macula. There is what appears to be a collection of large epithelial cells (Figure 5) on the thin membrane near the point of this
adhesion. This was first thought to be an artifact of sectioning,
but a similar area is seen in the opposite ear, which would suggest that this represents a real change in the saccule membrane.
The macula has a few very large polyhedral otoliths on its surface.

The utricle and the semicircular canals show no changes (Figure 6). The endolymphatic duct and sac (Figure 7) are lined with
epithelium lacking the usual convolutions seen in the adult but
otherwise appear normal.

The left ear shows fewer changes than the right (Figure 8). In
the cochlea, Reissner's membrane is not collapsed (Figure 9).
The position of Reissner's membrane and the stria vascularis
appear normal in the upper basal turn. Throughout much of its
length, however, the external attachment of Reissner's membrane is pulled toward the basilar membrane, rolling up the outer

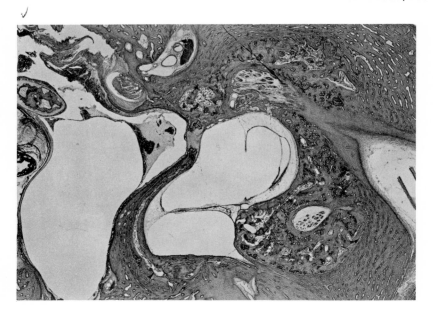

Figure 4

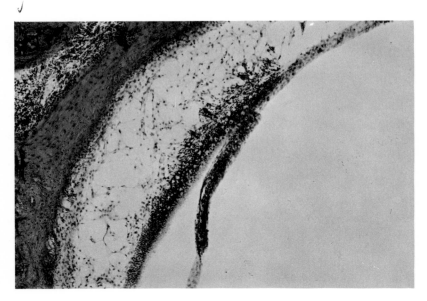

Figure 5

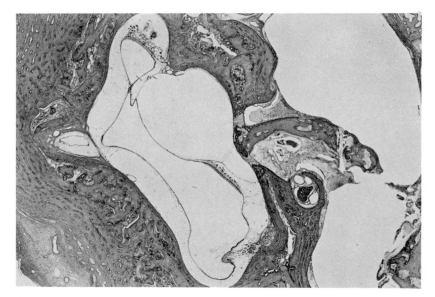

Figure 6

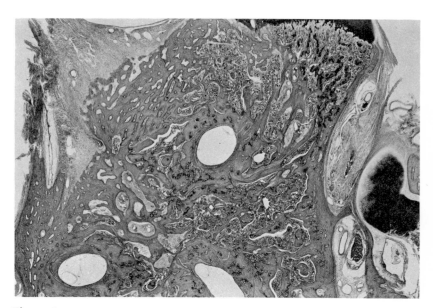

Figure 7

margin of the stria vascularis. There are a number of what appear to be cystic areas seen under the outer portion of the stria vascularis. The largest area (Figure 10) is seen in the extreme basal turn. Here the stria is raised and the outer attachment of Reissner's membrane appears to be pulling free. Perhaps this is the mechanism that eventually causes the detachment of the outer margin of the stria vascularis.

In this ear, the stria vascularis appears filled with capillaries and is of normal size. The tectorial membrane appears thinned and stretched but is in normal position. The organ of Corti appears normal, as do the internal and external sulci. Nerve fibers are plentiful and the spiral ganglion is normal. No abnormalities have been found in the blood vessels around the scala media.

The saccule is partially collapsed (Figure 11). The membranous portion (Figure 12) opposite the macula is thickened in the same manner as that seen in the opposite ear. A portion of the membrane appears stuck to the macula. Eosin staining in this region suggests a small scar between the membrane and the macula. The utricle appears normal (Figure 13), except for a few large dark-staining otoliths. The crista and macula appear normal.

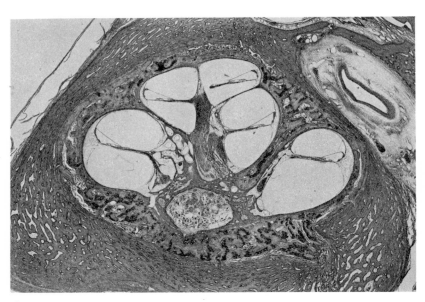

Figure 8

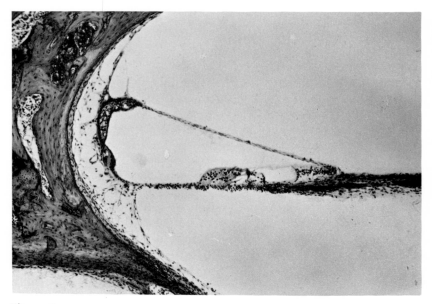

Figure 9

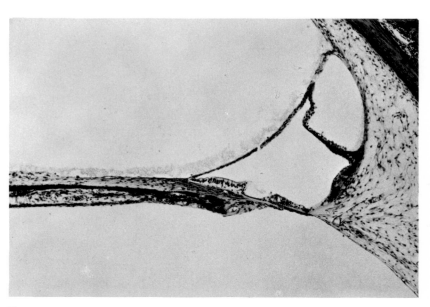

Figure 10

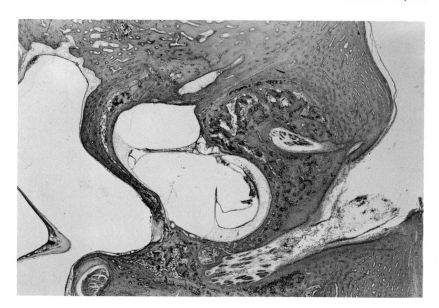

Figure 11

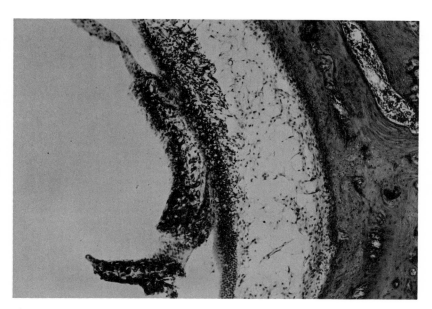

Figure 12

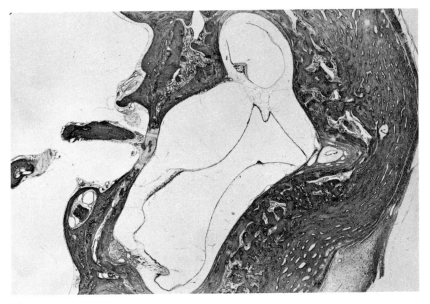

Figure 13

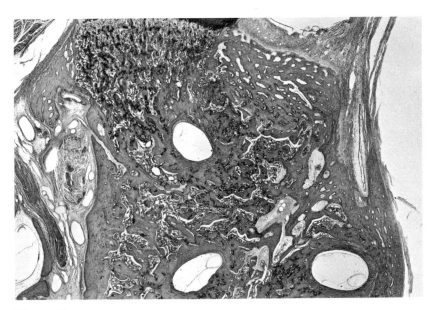

Figure 14

There is no evidence of collapse of its membrane. The semicircular canals are normal.

The endolymphatic duct and sac (Figure 14) are of the single-channel type with normal lining.

These ears appear to have undergone changes similar to those previously described by Carruthers, Nager, Lindsay, and others. In addition to the injuries described by these authors, the ears exhibit some additional changes worthy of reemphasis. The damage appears more marked in one ear—the right. There are cystic areas seen in the left ear which appear to unseat the outer end of the stria vascularis and the insertion of Reissner's membrane. In both ears a cellular thickening is present on the membranous portion of the saccule opposite the macula. In reviewing these saccular changes, Dr. Stacy Guild has compared them with the Tegmentum Vaculosum seen in birds.

It has become apparent in this study that prenatal rubella can damage a child while giving no clinical symptoms in the mother. Cultural and serological studies have demonstrated dramatically in these 79 children that much diagnostic information must in the future come from the virus laboratories. The morbidity of this infection during prenatal life is very severe, especially in those children exhibiting positive virus cultures.

This is but a preliminary report; much more information will be forthcoming as all the children under observation are tested and as the follow-up period reveals the accuracy of our test-retest, techniques for determination of hearing defects and our tests for the evaluation of developmental retardation. The significance of microcephaly must also be assessed. The two hundred-odd children suffering the stigmata of prenatal rubella, without culture or present serological evidence of the diseases, must have their hearing evaluated. Finally, a long term follow-up is necessary to study the cycle of the antibody titer rise and fall after rubella infection. More temporal-bone studies will be reviewed.

References

Alford, C. A., F. A. Neva, and T. H. Weller. 1964. "Virologic and Serologic Studies on the Human Products of Conception After Maternal Rubella." *New England J. Med.*, **271**:1275–1281.

Barr, B., and R. Lundström. 1961. "Deafness Following Maternal Rubella; Retrospective and Prospective Studies." *Acta oto-laryng.*, **53**:413–423.

Carruthers, D. G. 1945. "Congenital Deaf-Mutism as a Sequala of a Rubella-Like Maternal Infection During Pregnancy." *M. J. Australia*, **1**:315–320.

Goodhill, V. 1950. "Nerve Deaf Child: Significance of Rh, Maternal Rubella, and Other Etiologic Factors." *Ann. Otol. Rhin. & Laryng.*, **59**:1123–1147.

Gregg, N. M. 1941. "Congenital Cataract Following German Measles in the Mother." *Tr. Ophth. Soc. Australia*, **3**:35–46.

Hardy, J. B., G. R. Monif, and J. L. Sever. 1966. "Studies in Congenital Rubella, Baltimore 1964–1965. II. Clinical and Virologic." *Bull. Johns Hopkins Hosp.*, **118**:97–108.

Jackson, A. D. M., and L. Fisch. 1958. "Deafness Following Maternal Rubella: Results of a Prospective Investigation." *Lancet*, **2**:1241–1244.

Kamerbeek, A. E. H. M. 1949. "Het Rubella problem in het licht van Nederlandse Ervaringen." *Verhandl. van het Instituuit por praeventieve Geneskunde 14 Leiden.*

Lindsay, J. R., D. G. Carruthers, W. G. Hemenway, and M. S. Harrison. 1953. "Inner-Ear Pathology Following Maternal Rubella. "*Ann. Otol. Rhin. & Laryng.*, **62**:1201–1218.

Monif, G. R. G., J. G. Hardy, and J. L. Sever. 1966. "Studies in Congenital Rubella, Baltimore 1964–1965. I. Epidemiologic and Virologic." *Bull. Johns Hopkins Hosp.*, **118**:85–96.

Nager, F. R. 1952. "Microscopic Studies of Ears of Rubella Infants. *Pract. oto-rhino-laryng.*, **14**:337–359.

Parkman, P. D., E. L. Buescher, and M. S. Artenstein. 1962. "Recovery of Rubella Virus From Army Recruits." *Proc. Soc. Exper. Biol. & Med.*, **3**:225–230.

Schall, L. A., M. H. Lurie, and G. Kelemen. 1951. "Embryonic Hearing Organs After Maternal Rubella." Laryngoscope, **61**:99–112.

Sever, J. L., R. J. Huebner, G. A. Costallano, P. S. Sarma, A. Sabiyi, G. M. Schiff, and C. L. Cusumano. 1965. "Rubella Complement Fixation Test." Science, **148**(April 16):385–387.

Swan, C. 1944. "Congenital Malformation in Infants following Maternal Rubella during Pregnancy: Review of Investigations Carried Out in South Australia." *Tr. Ophth. Soc. Australia*, **4**:132–141.

Tondury, von G. 1951. "Zum Problem der Embryopathia Rubeolosa. Untersuchungen an menschlichen verschiedener Entwicklungestadien." *Bull. schweiz. Akad. med. Wissensch.*, **7**:307–325.

Tondury, von G. 1951. "Zum Problem der Embryopathia Rubeolosa." *Deutsche med. Wchnschr.*, **76**:1029–1030.

Weller, R. H., and F. A. Neva. 1962. "Propagation in Tissue Culture of Cytopathic Agents From Patients with Rubella-Like Illness." *Proc. Soc. Exper. Biol. & Med.*, **3**:215–225.

CONGENITAL DEAFNESS OF INFLAMMATORY ORIGIN

THE purpose of this study is to review the histopathology of a group of cases of acquired congenital deafness and to direct attention to features that appear to be characteristic of an inflammatory origin, either in fetal life or in early infancy.

Congenital deafness may result from a hereditary defect or may be acquired in fetal life or about the time of birth. The histopathology alone has often failed in the past to distinguish between the different types, partly because of the lack of a reliable history and partly because of similarities in the pathologic findings when the disorder had originated early in fetal life. A positive family history has in some instances indicated the probable hereditary nature of the defect, but a negative family history does not exclude a genetic relationship.

The discovery that maternal rubella might cause a hearing defect in the fetus along with other deformities was made after the epidemic in Australia and Tasmania more than twenty years ago. This was an important advance in the understanding of acquired congenital defects in the ear. The histopathologic examination of the inner ears affected by maternal rubella has revealed a consistent and distinctive pattern (Carruthers, 1945; Nager, 1952; Lindsay, et al., 1954).

The histopathological studies described in this paper were supported in part by grants from The Central Bureau of Research of the American Otological Society, Inc., Public Health Service Research Grant NB03358 and The Deafness Research Foundation.

Within the past few years clinical evidence of other etiologies for congenital deafness has been established, and the temporal bones from a few such cases have been obtained. The comparison of the histopathologic lesions in these ears with documented cases of deafness due to known viruses of mumps (Lindsay, et al., 1960) and measles (morbilli) (Lindsay, et al., 1954) in later childhood has revealed certain characteristics in common. The further examination of adult ears deafened during an acute upper respiratory infection of probable viral origin has further demonstrated similar characteristics (Beal, et al., to be reported). Further comparison with the lesions produced by certain other types of inner-ear disorders in fetal and adult life seem to establish certain histopathologic features as being characteristic of an inflammatory lesion of limited degree.

Maternal Rubella

The histopathologic characteristics of the inner ear defects due to maternal rubella have varied somewhat, apparently depending on the stage of fetal development at the time of the infection and probably also on the degree or severity of the inflammatory process. The ears from the well authenticated cases have shown degenerative process to have been limited to the cochlear duct and the structures within it, as well as the saccule, thereby constituting the so-called Scheibe type of deformity.

Case 1

This well documented case contributed by Carruthers of Australia to the University of Chicago laboratory illustrates features that appear to be characteristic.

The organ of Corti has varied in degree of degeneration but has been fairly well developed in some with hair cells recognizable. The stria vascularis has shown different degrees of atrophy. With advanced degeneration, a tendency to collapse of Reissner's membrane and reduction of the lumen of the cochlear duct has been observed.

A characteristic of the authenticated cases so far has been the retraction of the tectorial membrane toward the limbus where it has formed a globular mass covered by a membrane composed of a single layer of cells (Figure 1).

Degeneration of ganglion cells and nerve fibers has been relatively minor. The saccular wall was found collapsed onto the

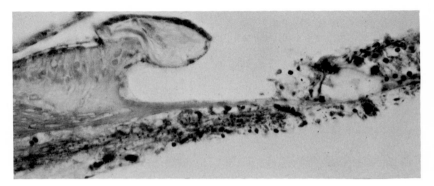

Figure 1. Photomicrograph of Corti's organ in Case 1 as it was found in the basal and middle coils in a documented case of deafness resulting from maternal rubella. Pillar cells and hair cells could be identified although distorted. The tectorial membrane was retracted to the limbus and covered by a cellular membrane.

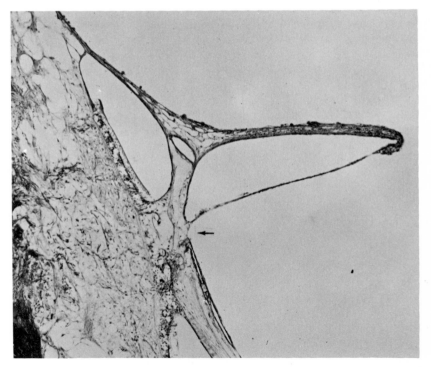

Figure 2. Photomicrograph of the saccule in Case 1. The macula showed irregular degeneration with post-inflammatory adhesions (arrow) between it and the saccular wall.

macula and in some cases adherent to degenerated areas of the sensory epithelium (Figure 2).

The perilymphatic spaces were free from any evidence of disease in these ears, hence the conclusion seemed warranted that the degenerative process had been due to invasion of the stria vascularis by the virus with inflammatory changes and secondary effects mainly on the tectorial membrane and the organ of Corti.

Endolymphatic Labyrinthitis and Neural Degeneration

Case 2

This second pair of ears (Ward, *et al.*, 1962) was obtained by Dr. Charles Kinney of Cleveland from a young adult severely deafened since birth or early infancy and processed and reported from the University of Chicago Laboratory presented similar characteristics but of different degree. The history in this case included a febrile illness at two months of age with high temperature, convulsions, and reputed nuchal rigidity, the total duration being 20 days. The pregnancy and delivery had been normal, and no deafness had been known in the preceding two generations. The essential features of the histopathology in these ears were the moderate degeneration of the stria vascularis, extensive degeneration of the organ of Corti, retraction of the tectorial membrane to the limbus with a covering by a single layer of cells. The spiral ganglion and the nerve fibers in the modiolus in this case showed extensive degeneration. The saccular wall had collapsed and was partly adherent to the macula (Figures 3 and 4).

This case illustrated some of the difficulties in differentiating a hereditary from an acquired deafness on the basis of the histopathology alone. The pathology differed from the known rubella cases in that there was more extensive degeneration of the organ of Corti and a corresponding reduction in ganglion cells and nerve fibers. Degeneration of nerve elements has been a characteristic of mild inflammatory reactions in the perilymphatic spaces but has, however, been found to a lesser degree in the known cases of viral labyrinthitis confined to the endolymphatic system. In this case, therefore, the absence of any evidence of an inflammatory process in the perilymphatic system seemed to indicate that the degeneration of nerve elements was related to the extensive degeneration of the organ of Corti. The appearance of the tectorial membrane corresponded to that seen in maternal rubella, mumps and measles (morbilli).

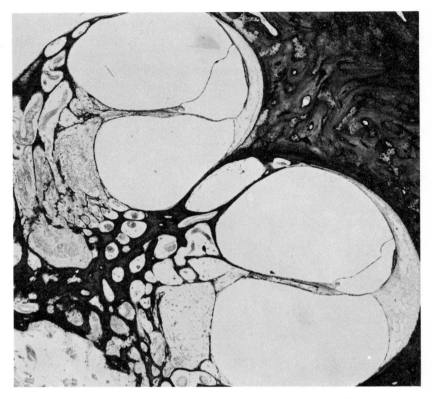

Figure 3. Case 2. Photomicrograph of a section through the basal and middle coils of the cochlea.

The spiral ganglion showed degeneration which was advanced in the basal coil and moderate in the middle and upper coils. The marked degeneration of Corti's organ, moderate degeneration of the stria vascularis and the retracted tectorial membrane, covered by a cellular membrane, are demonstrated.

The interpretation therefore seems warranted that this was a case of an acquired inflammatory reaction within the endolymphatic system corresponding to cases of known endolymphatic labyrinthitis of viral origin.

Meningogenic Labyrinthitis

Diffuse meningogenic labyrinthitis in infancy or early childhood has long been recognized as a cause for deaf-mutism.

The histopathology in diffuse labyrinthitis has been well documented in the European laboratories. Bilateral diffuse labyrinthi-

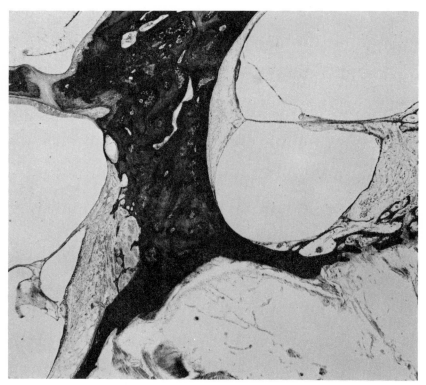

Figure 4. Case 2. Photomicrograph of a section through the basal coil and the saccule to demonstrate the degenerative changes of the saccule, the spiral ganglion and peripheral nerve fibres, Corti's organ and the stria vascularis.

tis has frequently caused a severe or total loss of hearing and vestibular function. The etiologic agent has usually been bacterial. Invasion of the labyrinths has occurred both by way of the middle ear air-cell systems or by way of the meninges. Previous to the development of chemotherapy and antibiotics a meningogenic bacterial labyrinthitis which survived was usually caused by the meningococcus, and loss of inner-ear function was often total.

Now that bacterial meningitis caused by pneumococcus, streptococcus, and staphyloccous has frequently been cured, the treatment has sometimes been too late to prevent total destruction of inner-ear function because of extension of the infection from the meninges.

A meningogenic labyrinthitis caused by invasion of the measles virus in meningoencephalitis has also been recorded (Nager, 1917) and has probably accounted for many cases of deaf-mutism.

The history obtained later in life may fail to indicate the time of onset of the deafness.

The degree of damage to the inner ear by meningogenic extension varies from unilateral hearing impairment to bilateral total loss of function. Two examples are presented to illustrate the latter type.

Case 3

Temporal bones contributed to the University of Chicago laboratory by Dr. Tapia of Chicago (detailed report to be published later).

This 82-year-old male was known to have been totally deaf since early childhood. There was no history of his having had meningitis in infancy.

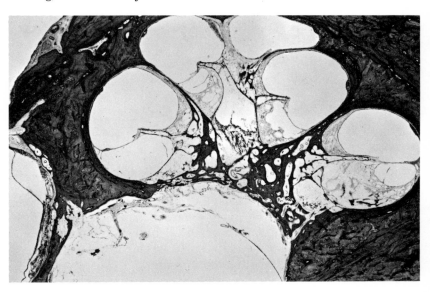

Figure 5. Case 3. Photomicrograph of a midmodiolar section of the cochlea of one ear. This illustrates proliferation of fibrous connective tissue in the scala vestibule and the scala tympani with irregular bone formation in the basal coil.

The scala media has been greatly dilated, the basilar membrane degenerated and displaced downwards, and Corti's organ and the stria vascularis almost totally degenerated. There has been subtotal degeneration of the peripheral cochlear neuron.

The degenerated saccule is also illustrated.

Both inner ears in this case show a similar type of pathologic picture.

There was a more or less diffuse hyperplastic reaction with fibrous tissue and bone formation throughout the perilymphatic system with obliteration of semicircular canals by bone and an extensive hydrops of the cochlear duct (Figures 5 and 6). In both

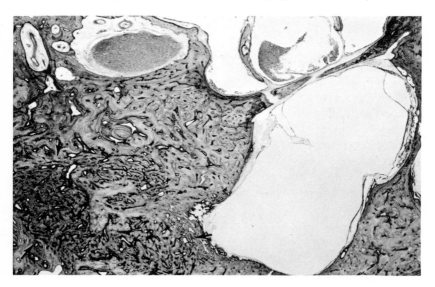

Figure 6. Case 3. Photomicrograph of a section through the vestibule at the level of the lower edge of the stapes footplate. The degenerated saccule is shown at the right. Other membranous structures within the vestibule have been destroyed.

The lumens of the semicircular canals have been filled by new bone (arrows) mostly lamellar and easily distinguished from the enchondral bony layer of the labyrinth capsule. The endosteal layer of bone which surrounds the canals has been partly resorbed and replaced by extensions of the new bone along vascular channels, thereby masking the exact outline of the former borders of the canals.

ears the endolymphatic aqueduct was involved in the hyperplastic process and the duct and sac reduced to remnants only.

The perilymphatic aqueduct and the closely related vein were open wide on one side, with the scala tympani at that region free from hyperplastic changes. In the other ear there was extensive new bone in the lower end of the scala tympani and blockage of the perilymphatic aqueduct.

There was almost total degeneration of the spiral ganglion and

Scarpas ganglion as well as the nerve fibers. Also, the organ of Corti was destroyed, and only small remnants of the stria vascularis and the tectorial membrane remained. The histopathologic findings in this case are therefore to be explained as an extension to the inner ear of a meningeal infection, probably caused by the meningococcus. A direct extension from a viral meningoencephalitis could also produce a perilymphatic labyrinthitis and therefore could not be definitely excluded in this case.

Case 4

This case was that of a 47-year-old adult with a history of having been totally deaf in her left ear and to have had only questionable remnants of hearing in the right since early childhood. History states that she had meningitis and brain fever at one year of age, the illness lasting six months. "Epilepsy" began at the age of four years. Death followed an injury from a fall during a convulsive seizure.

The middle ears were not remarkably abnormal.

The left ear showed obliteration of the cochlea by ossification and subtotal obliteration of the vestibular labyrinth (Figure

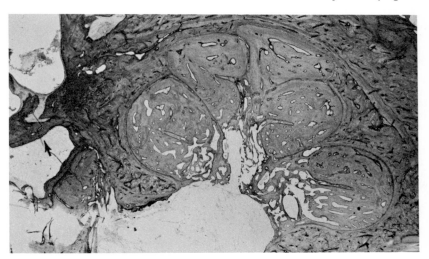

Figure 7. Case 4. Photomicrographs of a midmodiolar section of the left cochlea showing the almost complete ossification of the fluid spaces and absence of neural elements. The endosteal bone surrounding the fluid spaces is still recognizable as well as the bony spiral lamina.

The stapes has been fixed by new bone which party filled the vestibule (arrow).

7). The right ear showed the same type of destruction but less extensive obliteration by new bone. The eighth nerve was completely degenerated on both sides. These ears therefore represent a more extensive destructive process with obliteration of the membranous labyrinth and the sensory receptors due to meningogenic meningitis, most likely of meningococcal origin.

Comment

The four cases described represent types of acquired deafness either in fetal life or early childhood which present histopathology characteristic of inflammatory disease. In the first two cases the invasion of the cochlear duct and saccule has probably been through the bloodstream in the course of a viremia while the latter two represent a meningogenic invasion of the perilymphatic system by either a viral or bacterial agent.

In some instances, however, the histopathology alone may not provide for a definite differentiation between inherited and acquired changes. The next case may serve as an illustration.

Case 5

Male, age 18. Documentation and temporal bones sent by Dr. Patricia Davey of Sydney, Australia.

This child was considered to have normal hearing until 16 months of age, when he contracted measles and was noted by the parents to be deaf thereafter.

Both temporal bones showed a bony type of deformity of the labyrinths known as the Mondini Type (Figure 8) consisting of maldevelopment of the bony modiolus, absence of the interscalar septum between middle and apical coils, deformities of the cochlear duct, and grossly enlarged endolymphatic duct and sac.

There were also degenerative changes involving the organ of Corti in the basal coil and in part of the apical coil which presented features that were more suggestive of an inflammatory than of a developmental origin (Figures 9 and 10).

These consisted of degeneration of the organ of Corti, the stria vascularis and the tectorial membrane in the basal coils and a localized region in the apical coil which showed the tectorial membrane retracted into a semiglobular mass covered by a membrane composed of a single layer of cells.

Previous investigations have revealed variations of the Mondini

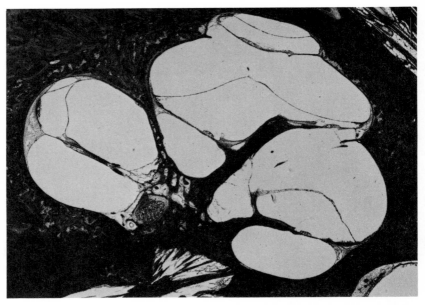

Figure 8. Photomicrograph of a midmodiolar section of the right cochlea. This demonstrates the maldevelopment of the modiolus which appeared only as a narrow column of bone above the basal coil. The absence of interscalar septa between the middle and basal coils and the deformity of the cochlear duct and its contents in the middle coil are evident.

type of deformity of the inner ears, with hearing varying from the normal to a marked impairment.

The history in this case was not sufficiently reliable to establish the time of onset of the deafness. Certain features of the histopathology involving the organ of Corti and the tectorial membrane were compatible with an inflammatory origin and bore a silirality to those found in certain cases of known viral disease (Lindsay, *et al.*, 1954, 1960). The combination of history and findings suggests rather strongly a Mondini type of developmental deformity as sufficient to explain the functional impairment.

The cases illustrating a meningogenic invasion of the labyrinths are characteristic in that they illustrate invasion of the perilymphatic spaces following the nerves and vessels in the modiolus as well as along the perilymphatic aqueduct. A viral meningo-encephalitis may apparently also invade the inner ears by these routes (Nager, 1907). Meningococcus meningitis, however, is also known to have been a common cause of acquired total loss of

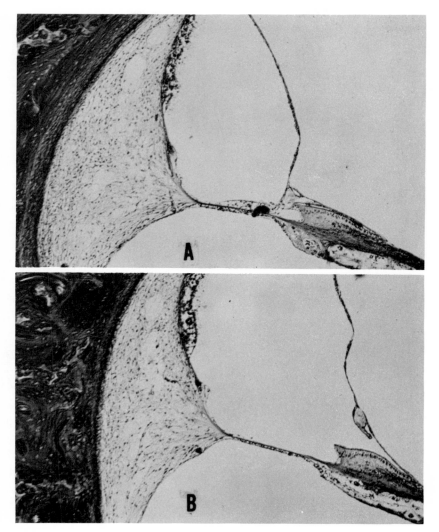

Figure 9. Case 5. Composite microphotograph of the basal coil at two adjacent areas. At level A there has been partial degeneration of Corti's organ and retraction of the tectorial membrane which has been incorporated in scar tissue between Reissner's membrane and Corti's organ.

At level B, Corti's organ was completely absent, nerve fibers to the region were absent, and the tectorial membrane retracted into a globular mass, surrounded by a cellular membrane and in contact with Reissner's membrane.

function of both labyrinths by destruction of soft tissue components and replacement by bone.

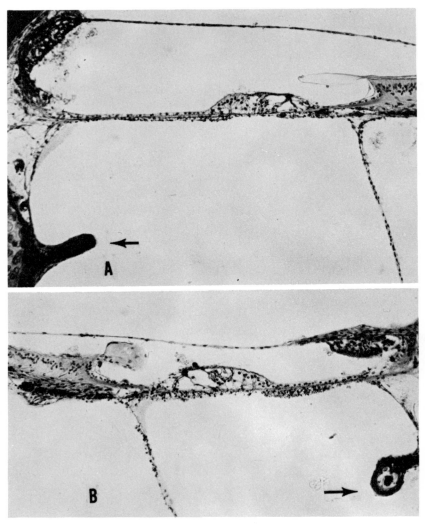

Figure 10. Case 5. Composite photomicrograph of the cochlear duct of the apical coil on the right side at two levels.

At level A nearest the apex Corti's organ, the tectorial membrane and the stria vascularis are shown to have been approximately normal.

At level B, about one half turn below level A, the stria vascularis is shown in an abnormal position, Corti's organ shows a normal development with some degeneration of hair cells but a normal complement of nerve fibers. The tectorial membrane appears retracted to the limbus and covered by a cellular membrane.

The documented cases of maternal rubella deafness have demonstrated features also observed in the ears damaged by measles (morbilli) and mumps, processed in our laboratory, and are believed to be indicative of a viremic invasion of the pars inferior of the labyrinth (cochlear duct and saccule) and in some instances (Lindsay, et al., 1954) also the pars superior.

Certain of these features, notably the changes within the cochlear duct, have also been found in other types of mild inflammatory reaction within the endolymphatic system and are therefore not specific for a viral endolymphatic labyrinthitis. They appear to be indicative of a mild inflammation which has produced degenerative changes of varying degree but which have not excited a hyperplastic response. These features have been characteristic in cases of endolymphatic labyrinthitis of known viral etiology in our series, as well as in two cases of deafness due apparently to an upper respiratory tract virus and which will be reported from the University of Chicago laboratory.

References

Beal, David D., Patricia R. Davey, and J. R. Lindsay (to be reported). "Inner-Ear Pathology of Congenital Deafness."

Carruthers, D. G. 1945. "Congenital Deaf-Mutism as a Sequela of a Rubella-Like Maternal Infection During Pregnancy." *M. J. Australia*, **32/1**:315–320.

Lindsay, J. R., D. G. Carruthers, M. S. Harrison and W. G. Hemenway. 1954. "Inner Ear Pathology in Children Following Maternal Rubella." *Ann. Otol. Rhin. & Laryng.*, **62**:461–464.

Lindsay, J. R., Patricia R. Davey, and P. H. Ward. 1960. "Inner-Ear Pathology in Deafness Due to Mumps." *Ann. Otol. Rhin. & Laryng.*, **69**:918–835.

Lindsay, J. R., and W. G. Hemenway. "Inner-Ear Pathology Due to Measles." *Ann. Otol. Rhin. & Laryng.*, **63**:754–771.

Nager, von F. R. 1907. "Beitrage zur Histologie der erworbenen Taubstummheit." *Ztschr. Ohrenh.*, **54**:217.

Nager, von F. R. 1952. "Histologische Ohruntersuchungen bei Kindern nach mütterlicher Rubella." *Pract. oto-rhino-laryng.*, **14**:337–360.

Ward, Paul H., Charles E. Kinney, and John R. Lindsay. 1962. "Inner Ear Pathology in Congenital Deafness." *Laryngoscope*, **72**(April):435–455.

CHAPTER **11** JOSEPH E. HAWKINS, JR.

IATROGENIC TOXIC DEAFNESS
IN CHILDREN

THE phenomenon of ototoxic deafness must be at least as old as the use of wormseed and Peruvian bark in the pre-Columbian pharmacopaeia of the Americas. Unfortunately, the documentation from that high and far-off time is scanty at best, and the names of the shamans who first remarked on the evil influence of chenopodium oil and cinchona alkaloids on their patients' hearing are lost in the dawn mists of prehistory.

Although salicylate ototoxicity is presumably more recent, it too is of a respectable antiquity. Schwabach (1884) writes of the disturbance of hearing caused by salicylic acid and quinine as "eine so allgemeine Thatsache" that it might seem to his readers superfluous to discuss it further. The mechanism of their action, incidentally, is not much better understood now than it was in Schwabach's day.

The tinnitus and hearing loss produced by these venerable drugs are variable and usually transitory. Full recovery is not unusual, as recorded by Schwabach, and as described by Roth (1918) in the case of chenopodium. It has remained for this generation to develop, by a sort of negative serendipity, therapeutic agents of highly specific, permanent ototoxic effect. These are the basic antibiotics, which began to appear some twenty years ago with the advent of streptomycin, and which now constitute a small antisocial family, of which the most objectionable junior members, at least from the point of view of hearing conservation, are neomycin and kanamycin.

156

With the widespread and perhaps not always wise clinical use of these antibiotics, drug ototoxicity is now firmly established as a cause of sensorineural deafness and is sufficiently common to warrant continued serious discussion and concern. This is the only form of deafness that is invariably iatrogenic. The physician therefore bears an extra heavy responsibility and must on occasion make exceedingly difficult decisions in choosing an antibiotic, for the ototoxic antibiotics can be invaluable weapons for him in life-threatening situations, and sometimes bacterial resistance leaves him little choice. It is essential that the physician, and especially the pediatrician, be aware of the risks as well as the stakes, and that he use these agents with full recognition that, while he may be saving the patient's life, he may also be destroying his hearing and his livelihood.

Streptomycin

The predilection of streptomycin for the vestibular neuroepithelium has often been stressed since its earliest use at the Mayo Clinic, announced by Hinshaw and Feldman in 1945. This vestibulotoxic effect is of greater danger to elderly patients than to the young, with their enviable powers of compensation and recovery. It is important to note, however, that the cortitoxic effect of streptomycin may be the more prominent in infants. Székely and Draskovich (1965) report from Budapest that when they tested 84 children 6 to 8 years of age who had received streptomycin in infancy, 43 had measurable elevation of threshold for high frequencies, whereas only 14 showed evidence of residual vestibular damage. These authors urge caution in using streptomycin in infants, since they are not able to report the initial symptoms of ototoxicity for themselves.

Streptomycin can and occasionally does cross the placental barrier in sufficient concentration to damage the fetal ear. Robinson and Cambon (1964) found 2 cases (out of 300 cases of hearing impairment in preschool children (in which the loss could clearly be attributed to streptomycin treatment of the mother. In one case, streptomycin had been given in a dose of 1 gm twice weekly between the 6th and 14th weeks of pregnancy. When the child was 4 years old, a severe, bilateral sensorineural loss was found, and caloric responses were absent. Impaired hearing had already been suspected at 6 months. In the second case, the mother received streptomycin 1 gm twice weekly during the last 4 months of pregnancy. At 2$^{1}/_{2}$ years the child walked with a broad base, had no speech and no hearing. Caloric responses were absent, and audiometry showed a flat sensorineural loss of 80 dB. In neither case was there any indication that the defect was genetically determined. Conway and Birt (1965) have reported minor residual disturbances of function in 8 of 17 children whose mothers received streptomycin during pregnancy. In 6 of them no caloric response was elicited, and in 4 there were audiometric changes, although not involving the speech frequencies. In two instances both the mother and the child showed a loss at 800 cps and reduced vestibular responses.

Neomycin

This is the most actively cortitoxic and nephrotoxic antibiotic known. Its use by the parenteral route is rarely if ever justified. Hubmann (1965) reports a case of right nephrectomy with normal renal function in which 5 gm of neomycin was given parenterally over a 6-day period covering the operation. One week later there was tinnitus, and after 14 days almost total loss of hearing, of course without recovery.

It is not always realized that neomycin can also be absorbed from the gut, the pleura, the peritoneum and from open wounds in sufficient concentration to cause renal failure and deafness. Greenberg and Momarz (1965) report the disastrous effects of oral neomycin in a 53-year-old woman operated on for a sigmoid diverticulum. She received 9 gm neomycin by mouth before the operation and 37 gm over a 3-week period after the operation. One week later she complained of tinnitus, and after two weeks she was totally deaf, although she had had no previous hearing difficulty. This loss was associated with acute renal failure, with a urine output of less than 300 ml per day.

A third case of neomycin deafness, still unpublished, I am permitted to mention through the courtesy of F. M. Jenkins, M.D., Resident in Otolaryngology at Washington University and the St. Louis VA Hospital. It is that of a 57-year-old arteriosclerotic patient with bilateral groin abcess following vascular surgery. He received continuous irrigation with 1 percent neomycin solution for 58 days, at which time he complained of difficulty in hearing. Three days later he was completely deaf. His wound is well healed, but his hearing is gone without a trace.

These cautionary tales deal with adults rather than children, but there is no reason to believe that children's ears are any less susceptible to neomycin used with such a free hand. Unfortunately, a recent monograph on poisoning compiled by a pediatrician contains the following terse rubric concerning both neomycin and kanamycin: "Oral or topical use is harmless. Intramuscular use should not exceed 10 days." (Arena, 1963.)

Kanamycin

With regard to kanamycin, the present picture is distinctly brighter, although it still belongs in the dangerous drug category, at least so far as hearing is concerned. Pediatric enthusiasm for kanamycin is high because of its remarkable effectiveness in coliform infections, gram-negative septicemia, and meningitis in the newborn, but that enthusiasm now appears to be tempered by a realization of its ototoxic potential. In 1962, Yow, Tengg, Bangs, Bangs, and Stephenson found 5 children who had suffered severe hearing loss among 30 who had received treatment with kanamycin, some of them in doses as large as 100 mg/kg, and for as long as 95 days. Dr. Martha Yow (1966) now recommends a dose not to exceed 10 to 15 mg/kg, for no longer than 10 days. She has seen excellent therapeutic results with no evidence of auditory complications when this schedule is followed. In the very young, however, auditory complications are not easy to detect, and one may hope that long-term follow-up studies of hearing will be made in children receiving kanamycin as infants. There is the unpleasant possibility that kanamycin may do subliminal damage to the organ of Corti which could manifest itself later as an enhanced susceptibility to further ototoxic or acoustic insult. The pediatrician who is concerned with the conservation of hearing should keep such a possibility, however remote it may be, in mind when he considers using kanamycin. In premature infants the additional hazard to hearing because of their inadequate renal function should not be forgotten.

Ototoxicity Studies in Laboratory Animals

The effects of kanamycin in laboratory animals have been described by a number of authors (e.g., Hawkins, 1959 a,b; Ward and Fernández, 1961; Darrouzet and de Lima Sobrinho, 1962), who used conventional histological methods to demonstrate the lesion in the organ of Corti. Similar lesions have been described in human ears, by Benitez, Schuknecht and Brandenburg (1962), Igarashi and Yoshinoba (1963), Jörgensen and Rotwitt-Schmidt (1963), and Matz, Wallace, and Ward (1965). Both in animals and in man, the outer hair cells appear to be the major site of damage, but the inner hair cells are not necessarily spared. Hawkins and Engström (1963), Engström and Kohonen (1965), Hawkins, Beger, and Aran (1965), and especially Kohonen in his dissertation (1965) have demonstrated the patterns of hair-cell and pillar-cell loss in kanamycin-treated guinea pigs by means of longitundinal or surface preparations (Figures 1, 2). There are marked similarities

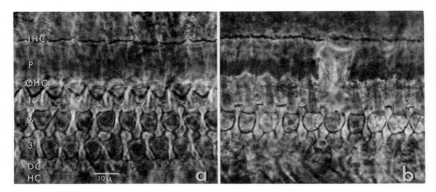

Figure 1. a. Longitudinal or surface preparation of normal organ of Corti of guinea pig, showing the mosaic pattern of the reticular lamina, with inner hair cells (IHC), tops of pillar cells (P) covering the tunnel, and three rows of outer hair cells (OHC). The stereocilia of IHC and row-1 OHC (W-patterns) are in focus. Between the OHC of row 1 are the paddle-shaped phalangeal processes ("Aussenruder") of the outer pillars, and between the OHC of rows 2 and 3 are the phalangeal processes of row-1 and -2 Deiters cells. DC, phalangeal processes of the row-3 Deiters cells; HC, Hensen cells. (3rd coil, 0s0₄ fixation, phase contrast.)

b. Longitudinal preparation of organ of Corti of kanamycin-treated guinea pig, showing destruction of row-1 OHC, leaving only phalangeal processes of outer pillars. One of the pillars is also missing. Row-2 OHC are represented by empty frames. In row 3 some cells are still present, but they are swollen and probably no longer functional. At the bottom of the picture, the processes of the third row Deiters cells can be seen. (KM, 200 mg/kg daily for 20 days, sacr. 3 days later, 3rd soil, 0s0₄ fixation, phase contrast.)

between the kanamycin lesion and that produced by acoustic trauma, save in this respect: Although all three rows of outer hair cells disappear from the basal portion of the organ of Corti after kanamycin treatment, higher up it is the cells of the first row that are most often damaged or missing. With acoustic trau-

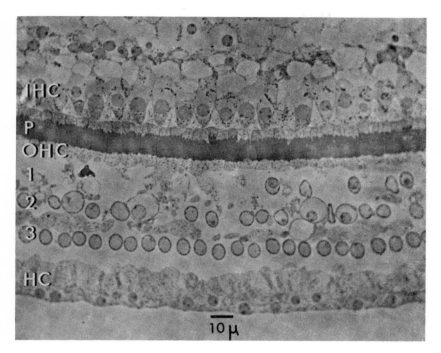

Figure 2. Selective destruction of the outer hair cells (OHC) of row-1 by kanamycin, longitudinal section, ca. 1μ, cut parallel to basilar membrane. Note that few OHC are present in row 1. Some are swollen and others are missing in row 2, whereas all are present and of normal diameter in row 3. The inner hair cells (IHC), pillar cells (P), and Hensen cells (HC) in this region are intact. (Guinea pig, KM 400 mg/kg daily for 8 days, sacr. 8 days later; 1st coil, OsO$_4$ fixation, araldite embedding, basic fuchsin stain, phase contrast.)

ma, on the other hand, it is the cells of the third row that disappear first (Hawkins, 1965). There is no obvious reason for this difference, but it is the smaller, shorter hair cells that seem to be most susceptible to kanamycin, i.e., those of the most basal region and those of the first row. In acoustic trauma, selective loss of the longer third-row cells may be related to the breaking of intercellular junctions between the Deiters and Hensen cells, as described by Beagley (1965).

Ultrastructural changes in the hair cells after kanamycin have been studied in the guinea pig by Duvall and Wersäll (1963) and by Farkashidy, Black, and Briant (1963), and in the fowl otocyst by Friedmann and Bird (1961). These authors have described early damage to stereocilia and to subcuticular mitochondria, with accumulation of osmiophilic material and formation of myelin figures. We have recently noted the disappearance of the characteristic parietal membranes in some outer hair cells. A more striking finding is marked loss of cells from the spiral ligament in the region behind the spiral prominence (Figure 3).

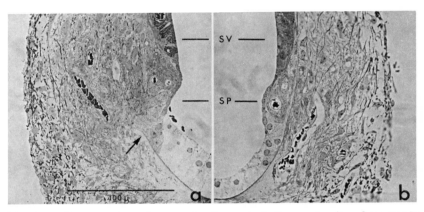

Figure 3. Degenerative changes in the spiral ligament after kanamycin. a) Normal guinea pig, b) kanamycin-treated (400 mg/kg for 8 days, as in fig. 2). In a) the arrow indicates the so-called root cells of the epithelium of the outer sulcus, which send long, branching processes far into the connective tissue of the ligament. In b) note the shrunken cells and loss of substance of the spiral ligament. Although the stria vascularis (SV), spiral prominence (SP), and other epithelial structures look normal, some of the long processes of the root cells have disappeared, leaving gaps and lacunae, especially near capillaries. (OsO$_4$ fixation, araldite embedding, 1μ sections, basic fuchsin stain).

Present evidence suggests that it may be the distal extensions and branches of the so-called root cells of the outer sulcus, first described by Prenant (1892) and Retzius (1893), that are affected. Whether their disappearance precedes the damage to outer hair cells or is concurrent with it remains to be determined, but we must recognize the possibility that degeneration of the outer hair cells may not be the primary kanamycin lesion after all.

We have seen no such clear-cut effects on the stria vascularis in these animals, although various authors from Rüedi (1951) to Müsebeck and Schätzle (1963) have concluded that the primary damage may be there. Our present view is that kanamycin reaches the organ of Corti by way of the inner and outer spiral vessels beneath the basilar membrane, which appear, from our own anatomical studies and from the recent occlusion experiments of Lawrence (1966), to furnish its terminal blood supply (Figure 4).

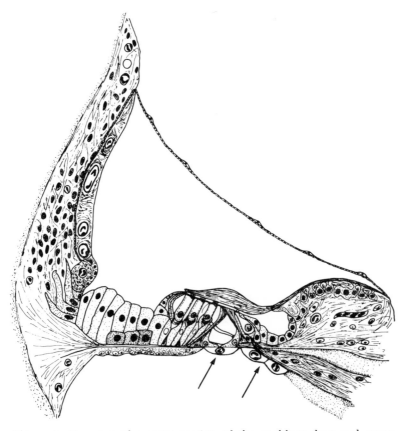

Figure 4. Drawing of a cross-section of the cochlear duct and organ of Corti. The arrows point to the outer and inner spiral vessels beneath the tunnel and the inner hair cells and inner sulcus. These capillaries furnish the terminal blood supply to Corti's organ. (Guinea pig, 1st coil).

Changes that we have seen in the spiral ligament may be related also to the tendency of antibiotics to attain a somewhat higher concentration in the perilymph than in the cerebrospinal fluid and to persist there, as demonstrated by Vrabec, Cody, and Ulrich (1965). This concentration effect may be related to binding of the antibiotic by protein in the perilymph.

Two Forms of Ototoxicity

Present experimental evidence as well as clinical observations of long standing strongly indicate that the ototoxic effects of quinine and salicylates are essentially different from those of the basic antibiotics. Recovery of hearing loss after quinine and salicylate intoxication is common, whereas after kanamycin treatment it is virtually unknown. Our preliminary experiments with large single doses of sodium salicylate in the operant-conditioned monkey (Stebbins and Hawkins, 1966) show acute loss of about 20dB and prompt recovery (i.e., within 24 hours). Various authors have speculated about uncoupling of phosphorylations (Meyers, Bernstein, and Fostiropoulos, 1965) or changes in the tectorial membrane (McCabe and Dey, 1965) caused by salicylates, but in guinea pigs we have seen evidence of vasoconstriction in the stria vascularis (Figure 5) and partial blockage of the spiral vessels beneath the basilar membrane by swollen endothelial cells (Figure 6) after both sodium salicylate and quinine.

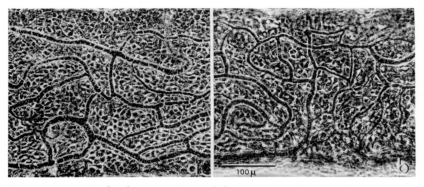

Figure 5. Longitudinal preparations of the stria vascularis: a) Normal guinea pig, and b) guinea pig sacrificed 30 minutes after a single dose of sodium salicylate, 500 mg/kg s.c. After salicylate the strial capillaries appear somewhat constricted and the perivascular spaces surrounding them are more easily seen. (1st coil, OsO_4 fixation, phase contrast.)

It is reasonable to infer that it is the resulting ischemia from which other changes may follow. Our findings therefore support the much older conclusion of Gradenigo (1892) and Wittmaack (1903) that the quinine effect on the ear is caused by vasoconstriction in the inner ear similar to the retinal ischemia that is readily observed in quinine-treated animals. On the other hand,

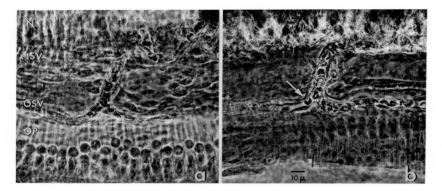

Figure 6. The spiral vessels (capillaries) beneath the basilar membrane: ISV, inner spiral vessel beneath the tympanic lip and inner hair cells. OSV, outer spiral vessel beneath tunnel of Corti. N, myelinated nerve fibers in osseous spiral lamina; OP, bases of outer pillars.

a. Normal guinea pig, 3rd coil, with typical well-filled capillary arches.

b. Guinea pig, 1st coil, sacrificed 65 min. after quinine dihydrochloride, 250 mg/kg, s.c. Note the partial occlusion of the left-hand capillary arch by the swollen endothelial cell (arrow), which is blocking the passage of a red blood cell. The right-hand capillary arch appears to be partly constricted, as shown by the wide perivascular space surrounding it. Partial occlusion and constriction were found in the spiral vessels throughout the cochlea after a large single dose of quinine or salicylate. (Longitudinal preparations, OsO₄ fixation, phase contrast.)

we have seen no clear evidence of hair-cell changes after acute quinine (250 mg/kg) and salicylate (500 mg/kg) intoxication similar to those pictured by Falbe-Hansen (1941) and by Rüedi (1951) after prolonged administration.

We may conclude that the salicylates, although an ever-present danger to children's lives through accidental or therapeutic poisoning (cf. Riley and Worley, 1956), are seldom if ever a threat to their hearing alone. The ototoxic antibiotics, on the other hand, are a threat to hearing, and a serious one, unless they are employed with the greatest circumspection and only in cases where no other antimicrobial agent will serve.

Acknowledgments

The author is indebted to Mrs. Estella N. Tennant for preparing the sections shown in Figs. 2 and 3, to Mrs. Jill Myerson and Mr. Jai Riu for the drawing in Fig. 4, and to Messrs. Max Tedford and Vernon Maulbetsch for expert photographic advice and processing of the photomicrographs.

Kanamycin sulfate (Kantrex®) was generously furnished by Dr. H. Leo Dickison of Bristol Laboratories, Syracuse, N. Y.

This work was supported by Public Health Service Research Grants NB 05065–03 and NB 05785–01A1 from the National Institute of Neurological Diseases and Blindness.

References

Arena, J. M. 1963. *Poisoning.* Springfield, Illinois: C. C Thomas.

Beagley, H. A. 1965. "Acoustic Trauma in the Guinea Pig. I. Electrophysiology and Histology." *Acta oto-laryng.*, **60**:437–451.

Benitez, J. T., H. F. Schuknecht, and J. H. Brandenburg. 1962. "Pathologic Changes in Human Ear After Kanamycin." *Arch. Otolaryng.*, **75**:192–197.

Conway, N., and B. D. Birt. 1965. "Streptomycin in Pregnancy: Effect on the Foetal Ear." *Brit. M. J.*, **5456**:260–263.

Darrouzet, J., and E. de Lima Sobrinho. 1962. "Oreille interne, kanamycine, et traumatisme acoustique: étude expérimentale." *Rev. laryng.*, **83**:781–806.

Duvall, A. J., and J. Wersäll. 1963. "Site of Action of Streptomycin Upon Inner Ear Sensory Cells." *Acta oto-laryng.*, **57**:581-598.

Engström, H., and A. Kohonen. 1965. "Cochlear Damage from Ototoxic Antibiotics." *Acta oto-laryng.*, **59**:171–178.

Falbe-Hansen, J. 1941. "Clinical and Histological Experimental Studies on Effects of Salicylate and Quinine on the Ear." *Acta oto-laryng.*, Suppl. 44.

Farkashidy, J., R. G. Black, and T. D. R. Briant. 1963. "Effect of Kanamycin on the Internal Ear: An Electrophysiological and Electron Microscopic Study." *Laryngoscope*, **73**:713–727.

Friedman, I., and E. S. Bird. 1961. "The Effect of Ototoxic Antibiotics and of Penicillin on the Sensory Areas of the Isolated Fowl Embryotocyst in Organ Culture: An Electron Microscopic Study." *J. Path. & Bact.*, **81**:81–90.

Gradenigo, G. 1892. "Die Krankheiten des Labyrinthes und des Hörnerven." *Handbuch der Ohrenheilkunde*, ed. by H. Schwartze, **2**:475–478. Leipzig: F. C. Vogel.

Greenberg, L. H., and H. Momarz. 1965. "Audiotoxicity and Nephrotoxicity Due to Orally Administered Neomycin." *J.A.M.A.*, **194**: 827–828.

Hawkins, J. E., Jr. 1959. "Antibiotics and the Inner Ear." *Tr. Am. Acad. Ophth.*, **63**:206–218.

Hawkins, J. E., Jr. 1959. "The Ototoxicity of Kanamycin." *Ann. Otol. Rhin. & Laryng.*, **68**:698–715.

Hawkins, J. E., Jr. 1965. "Cytoarchitecture of the Cochlear Transducer." *Cold Spring Harbor Symp. Quant. Biol.* **30**:147–157.

Hawkins, J. E., Jr., V. Beger, and J. M. Aran. 1965. "Antibiotic Insults to Corti's Organ." *Sensorineural Hearing Processes and Disorders*, ed. by A. B. Graham. Boston: Little, Brown & Co. (in press).

Hawkins, J. E., Jr., and H. Engström. 1964. "Effect of Kanamycin on Cochlear Cytoarchitecture." *Acta. oto-laryng. Suppl.*, **188**:100–106.

Hinshaw, H. C., and W. H. Feldman. 1945. "Streptomycin in Treatment of Clinical Tuberculosis: A Preliminary Report." *Proc. Staff Meet. Mayo Clin.*, **20**:313–318.

Hubman, R. 1965. "Irreversible Ertaubung nach Neomycinbehandlung bei normaler Nierenfunktion." *Der Urologe*, **4**:27–28.

Igarashi, M., and T. Yoshinoba. 1963. "Kanamycin Deafness: A Human Temporal Bone Report." *Oto-rhino-laryng. Clin. (Kyoto)*, **56**:301. Cit. *Excerpta Med. XI Oto-rhino-laryng.*, **17**:97.

Jenkins, F. M. 1966. Personal Communication.

Jorgensen, M. B., and M. Rotwitt-Schmidt. 1962. "The Ototoxic Effect of Kanamycin: A Clinical and Histological Study." *Acta oto-laryn.*, **55**:537–544.

Kohonen, A. 1965. "Effect of Some Ototoxic Drugs Upon the Pattern and Innervation of Cochlear Sensory Cells in the Guinea Pig." *Acta. oto-laryng.*, Suppl. 208.

Lawrence, M. 1966. "Effects of Interference with Terminal Blood Supply on Organ of Corti." *Laryngoscope* **76**:1318–1377.

McCabe, P. A., and F. L. Dey. 1965. "The Effect of Aspirin Upon Auditory Sensitivity." *Am. Otol.*, **74**:312–325.

Matz, G. J., T. H. Wallace, and P. H. Ward. 1965. "The Ototoxicity of Kanamycin." *Laryngoscope*, **75**:1690–1698.

Meyers, E. N., J. M. Bernstein, and G. Fostiropoulos. 1965. "Salicylate Ototoxicity; A Clinical Study. *New England J. Med.*, **273**:587–590.

Müsebeck, K., and W. Schätzle. 1962. "Experimentelle Studien zur Ototoxicität des Dihydrostreptomycins." *Arch. Ohren-Nasen-u. Kehlhopfh.*, **181**:41–48.

Prénant, A. 1892. "Recherches sur la paroi externe du limaçon des Mammifères et specialement sur la Strie vasculaire." Internat. Monatsschr. f. Anat. u. Physiol., **9**:6–36; **9**:41–75.

Retzius, G. 1893. "Über das Epithel des Sulcus spiralis cochleae." *Biol. Untersuchungen, n. F.*, **5**:39–40.

Riley, H. D., and L. Worley. 1956. "Salicylate Intoxication." *Pediatrics*, **18**:578–594.

Robinson, G. C., and K. G. Cambon. 1964. "Hearing Loss in Infants of Tuberculous Mothers Treated With Streptomycin During Pregnancy." *New England J. Med.*, **27**:949–951.

Roth, D. A. 1918. "Some Dangers of the Chenopodium Treatment." *South. M. J.*, **11**:733–734.

Rüedi, L. 1951. "Some Animal Experimental Findings on the Functions of the Inner Ear." *Ann. Otol. Rhin. & Laryng.*, **60**:993–1023.

Schwabach, D. 1884. "Ueber bleibende Störungen im Gehörorgan nach Chinin und Salicylgebrauch." *Deutsche med. Wchnschr.*, **10**:163–166.

Stebbins, W. C., and J. E. Hawkins, Jr. 1966. "A Behavioral Method for the Study of Ototoxicity in Non-Human Primates." Proc. U. S. Food and Drug Admin. Conf. on Non-Human Primate Toxicology, Wash. D. C., June 12–14 (to be published).

Székely, T., and E. Draskovich. 1965. "Die Wirkung der Streptomycins auf das Gehörorgan von Kleinkindern." *Ztschr. Laryng. Rhin. Otol.*, **44**:15–22.

Vrabec, D. P., D. T. R. Cody, and J. A. Ulrich. 1965. "A Study of the Relative Concentrations of Antibiotics in Blood, Spinal Fluid and Perilymph in Animals." *Ann. Otol. Rhin. & Laryng.*, **74**:688–705.

Ward, P. H., and Fernandez, C. 1961. "The Ototoxicity of Kanamycin in Guinea Pigs." *Ann. Otol., Rhin. & Laryng.*, **70**:132–142.

Wittmaack, K. 1903. "Beiträge zur Kenntniss der Wirkung des Chinins auf das Gehörorgan. *Pflügers Arch. ges. Physiol.*, **95**:209–233.

Yow, M. D., N. E. Tengg, J. Bangs, T. Bangs, and W. Stephenson. 1962. "The Ototoxic Effects of Kanamycin Sulfate in Infants and Children." *J. Pediat.*, **60**:230–242.

Yow, M. D. 1966. (Panel Discussion) "Kanamycin in Pediatric Practice With Special Reference to Observations on Ototoxicity." *Kanamycin: Appraisal After Eight Years of Clinical Application. Ann. New York Acad. Sc.*, **132**:1037-1044.

CATHERINE SMITH

DISCUSSION: PATHOLOGY

THE foregoing chapters contain many examples of pathology in the inner ear associated with deafness in children. Many points of clinical importance have been emphasized, such as Dr. Bordley's interesting finding that it was possible to obtain positive virus cultures even at four to six months after birth from some children with prenatal exposure to rubella. I will confine my comments to the pathological findings presented.

The cases and temporal bones described can be separated into three catetories: those with deafness of genetic origin; those with deafness acquired by pathogens and toxic materials transmitted in general to the ear by the blood stream; and those with deafness caused by meningogenic labyrinthitis.

Let us consider first the congenital pathology of genetic origin. As Dr. Schuknecht has pointed out, the development of the inner ear may be arrested at a number of stages. This may occur early, before differentiation of the epithelial primordium of the cochlear duct, or it may be late, as found in cases of partial deafness.

There are several well-known strains of animals with inherited inner-ear defects and with symptoms of auditory of vestibular disturbances, or both. Observations have been made on the Dalmatian dogs, white cats, and several strains of rodents. Such studies are of considerable value in giving us a better understanding of human genetic defects. In animals, the progression of changes in a number of siblings can be studied by application of several techniques and much useful information gained. One particularly thorough study was that of Bosher and Hallpike (1965) on the deaf white cat reported last year. Many of you are undoubtedly familiar with it, but I should like to go briefly over the findings there. One interesting facet was that they found, contrary to previous information, that the cat organ of Corti was not fully developed throughout at birth and that it did not attain its mature form until 14 to 21 days after birth. In the deaf cats, the lesion similar to the Scheibe type of degeneration was not manifest until the fifth postnatal day. The organ of Corti atrophied first, the stria vascularis later, and these changes were well advanced by 12 to 21 days. It was concluded that the defect was a dominant trait. Because it was unilateral in some animals and was not manifest at birth, it was felt that some environmental factors intervened. In other words, in some ears the degeneration was presumably prevented.

In a recent symposium on the embryopathic activity of drugs, Fauts (1965) has emphasized that the pharmacologic responses of the immature human (fetus and newborn) may differ greatly both quantitatively and qualitatively from those of the adult. Recent research has shown, for example, that several of the hepatic microsomal drug-metabolizing enzymes normally present in adults are absent or at low values in neonatal rabbits, guinea pigs, and mice.

If the maturing cell groups in early postnatal life demand some element that continues too long to be low in concentration, or if some metabolic system is defective and does not properly mature, this could explain Hallpike's "environmental factor" and late degeneration. Obviously, not only structural studies, but also histochemical and biochemical studies are in order.

Attention should also be given to the spiral ganglion and Scarpa's ganglion and to the central nervous system in hereditary conditions. Kikuchi and Hilding (1965) have recently found that the efferent olivo-cochlear nerve bundle is greatly reduced in size as well as delayed in its penetration to the cochlea in the Shaker-1 mouse. Whether this is due to a central deficiency or to a faulty inductive process is unclear. I would urge that an effort be made to find monkeys with hereditary defects so that these as well as lower animals might be studied.

It would be difficult to utilize cytological alteration as a criterion for judging the pathology due to viral infections and other infectious or toxic agents, because of the long time lapse between disease and acquisition of the temporal bones, sometimes an entire life span. As Dr. Hemenway has pointed out, virus infections are characterized by intracellular inclusion bodies. (Smith, et al., in preparation) have been studying the ultrastructural changes in respiratory epithelium during colds (where the infection is presumably viral) and find intracellular bodies in some epithelial cells. Others show enlarged mitrochondria and nuclear changes. These cellular alterations are visible within the first few days after onset of symptoms. Complete cellular disintegration follows quickly. By the end of one week, the cells are in such a complete stage of lysis that many are not even readily identifiable as epithelial cells. The process in the respiratory tract may be more rapid than in the ear because the cells are directly available to the airborne infectuous agent. Nevertheless, one would not expect to be able to find specific cell changes at a late date in viral labyrinthine infections but rather only complete degeneration. Some cell groups, however, may be more readily attacked and destroyed than others.

In this regard, it has been pointed out by Drs. Lindsay, Bordley, and Hemenway that many well-documented cases of viral deafness are characterized by degeneration of the stria vascularis, the organ of Corti, and the tectorial membrane. Saccular degeneration may also be present. Dr. Hemenway found moderate vestibular degeneration in one case, but in most, the vestibule was apparently normal. This picture is in contrast to the meningogenic invasion of the perilymphatic spaces described by Dr. Lindsay, where there was complete destruction of the membranous labyrinth.

Dr. Lindsay has suggested the former picture results from an invasion of the stria by the virus, with secondary effects on the organ of Corti and tectorial membrane. And this seems quite reasonable. The virus is apparently carried into the inner ear by means of the blood stream.

Let us look briefly at the small blood vessels of the cochlea. The capillaries are well organized into several distinct groups (Smith, 1954). Two of these are of particular interest here. One is the small plexus found in the spiral ligament just behind the spiral prominence. The other is the dense capillary network of the stria vascularis. This is a wide band of interconnecting capillaries, separated from the other capillaries of the spiral ligament, and situated within the epithelial layer.

Perlman and Kimura (1965) have observed that blood flow is

slower in the capillaries of the stria vascularis than in other capillaries of the spiral ligament. The reduced blood flow plus the intra-epithelial situation may permit a more rapid multiplication of the virus in the strial epithelium, with subsequent discharge into the endolymph. The changes in the tectorial membrane might be caused by alterations in the endolymph, direct effects on the limbus, or a combination of both.

This possibly could also explain why the vestibular labyrinth sometimes escapes damage, for there is no large, intra-epithelial capillary pool to be found in the vestibule. There are capillary plexuses beneath the maculae and cupulae, but these are not intra-epithelial, and their architecture does not suggest any unusual reduction of blood flow (Smith, 1953).

At the present time, the pathological characteristics of virus infections in the membranous labyrinth are not clearly defined, and the clinical history would seem to be a more important diagnostic aid. Experimental viral infections of the mammalian ear might also give us valuable information.

The question of the peculiar toxicity of streptomycin and related drugs to the inner ear has still not been satisfactorily answered, although Dr. Hawkins has given us some new findings. Two factors would seem to be most important: the special metabolic properties of the cells and the drug concentration in their immediate vicinity. It is possible that the concentration of the drugs is greater in the labyrinthine fluids than in other tissue fluids because of a rapid entry or slow elimination, or both. The drugs might also become concentrated in the gelatinous membranes (the tectorial membrane, the macular and cupular membranes) into which the hairs of the hair cells are inserted. A recent paper by Voldrich (1965) indicates that streptomycin may persist longer in the labyrinthine fluids than in the blood. Even though there may be a high drug concentration in the inner-ear fluids, the evidence also indicates that some metabolic characteristic of the hair cells is an important factor, for in low drug concentrations the hair cells are first to degenerate.

Dr. Hawkins's observations on changes in cells behind the spiral prominence in kanamycin-treated guinea pigs could be related to absorption of an endolymph with a high drug concentration. This region is one that has been frequently implicated in theories of exchange of materials between endolymph and the presumed perilymph in the spiral ligament. The distinct capillary plexus in the spiral prominence supports such theories.

There are many other important points brought out in the foregoing chapters that could be discussed, and I hope the authors will pardon me that I do not refer to them. The number of temporal bones available for study has remarkably increased in the past few years, and undoubtedly many new cases of inner-ear pathology will soon be added to those presented here. It is important to compare these findings with experimental studies in animals, where conditions are more readily controlled and studied, so that we may know more of the course and extent of the pathology of both congenital deafness as well as deafness acquired in early postnatal life.

References

Bosher, S. K., and C. S. Hallpike. 1965. "Observations on the Histological Features, Development and Pathogenesis of the Inner-Ear Degeneration of the Deaf White Cat." *Proc. Roy. Soc. (Sec. B)*, **162**: 147–190.

Fauts, J. R. 1965. "Metabolism of Drugs by the Fetus." *Symp. on Embryopathic Activity of Drugs*, edited by Robson, Sullivan and Smith. Boston: Little, Brown & Co.

Kikuchi, K., and D. A. Hilding. 1965. "The Defective Organ of Corti in Shaker-1 Mice." *Acta. oto-laryng.*, **60**:287–303.

Perlman, H., and R. Kimura. 1955. "Observations of the Living Blood Vessels of the Cochlea." *Ann. Otol., Rhin. & Laryng.*, **64**:1176–1192.

Smith, C. A. 1953. "The Capillaries of the Vestibular Membrane Labyrinth in the Guinea Pig." *Laryngoscope*, **63**:87–104.

Smith, C. A. 1954. "Capillary Areas of the Membranous Labyrinth." *Ann. Otol., Rhin. & Laryng.*, **63**:435–447.

Smith, C. A., W. T. K. Bryan, and M. P. Bryan. "Ultrastructural Change in Nasal Epithelial Cells During Colds" (in preparation).

Voldrich, L. 1965. "The Kinetics of Streptomycin, Kanamycin, and Neomycin in the Inner Ear." *Acta. oto-laryng.*, **60**:243–248.

PART **IV**

MEDICAL TREATMENT AND RESEARCH

THE GENETICS OF CHILDHOOD
DEAFNESS

CHILDHOOD deafness may be defined in many different ways. Through the use of audiometry, any arbitrary degree of deviation from a standard may be defined as deafness. In the absence of audiometric data, a wide variation in definition is possible, using less sophisticated and/or quantitative criteria.

Audiometric examinations are not available in most published studies and when available have not proved a good diagnostic criterion for causal factors (Fisch, 1955). Profound losses can usually be detected by the failure of the child to develop language, but these language development failures may indicate other conditions, such as general mental deficiency and difficulties with the speech mechanism itself. Less severe and unilateral defects may go undetected by physicians, and even by the affected individual, for long periods (Fraser, 1964).

Since genetic studies are usually based on the severe congenital loss group, as defined by the presence of the individual in the special schools for the deaf or by "deaf mutism" caused by lack of language development, genetic conclusions may be biased to some degree by these limitations of the data base. These limits are probably not a severe defect, however, compared with some of the other assumptions that must be made in genetic analyses of human data.

Estimation of the Prevalence of Childhood Deafness

Genetic analyses of human traits often presume knowledge of the prevalence of the trait in question. The recorded prevalences of deafness in various countries (Table I), even those with relatively good statistics, are generally recognized to be lower than

TABLE I

PREVALENCE OF DEAFNESS PER 100,000 POPULATION
(AFTER LUMIO AND PALJAKKA, 1964, WITH ADDITIONS)

	Year of Study	Prevalence
Chicago School Pupils—kdg.-grade 8 (Powers, 1964)	1964	160
Honduras	1935	138
Finland	1964	131
Japan (ages 5 to 39 years)	1947	118
Switzerland	1953	94
Scotland	1930	87
England-Wales	1930	85
Philippines (Santillan, **et al.**, 1965)	1965	83
New York State (Sank, 1963)	1960	80
Iceland	1948	76
India	1931	66
Canada	1941	63
Belgium	1950	59
Norway	1930	53
Union of South Africa (Whites)	1936	49
France	1946	47
U.S.A.—under age 5 (Beasley, 1940)	1936	46
Denmark	1946	45
N. Ireland	1956	45
Mexico (over age 12 years)	1940	39

the facts. On the other hand, the criteria for childhood deafness in the Chicago school data may be more inclusive than are usually used. A convenient intermediate prevalence estimate as used in the genetic analysis here is one per thousand. There is probably real variation in the prevalence of childhood deafness from country to country and population to population, but how much is not known.

Many observations about childhood deafness suggest that genetic factors are important in its etiology (Table II). An elevated

TABLE II

OBSERVATIONS SUGGESTING THAT GENETIC FACTORS PLAY
A ROLE IN THE ETIOLOGY OF A TRAIT (MORTON, 1962)

1. Elevated risk in relatives compared with the General population.
2. Greater concordance of the trait among identical than fraternal twins.
3. An excess of consanguinity among normal parents of trait possessors.
4. Failure of the trait to appear in unrelated individuals with high exposure to trait possessors.
5. Onset at a characteristic age without a known precipitating event.
6. Variation among populations and behavior in outcrossing in accordance with genetic theory.
7. Occurrence of homologous, inherited conditions in other mammals.

risk in relatives but not in unrelated contacts, increased consanguinity among parents, and increased concordance or agreement between pair members of identical as opposed to fraternal twins—all are true observations about childhood deafness. It is necessary to recognize, however, that these observations only suggest a genetic component in etiology but do not provide any information about the nature of the genetic mechanisms involved.

Twin Study of Deafness

Data on childhood deafness in twins (Table III), collected and evaluated by Sank (1963), show that identical twins have 59 percent concordance or similarity in regard to profound deaf-

TABLE III

STUDIES OF PROFOUND DEAFNESS IN TWINS (SANK, 1963)

Type of Twins	Concordant	Discordant	% Concordant
Monozygotic	10	7	59
Dizygotic	4	16	19
Total	14	23	

ness occurring before age 17 years. This degree of concordance is suggestive of a large genetic component in the etiology of deafness. The 19 percent concordance of fraternal twin pairs is expected when common environmental factors play a considerable etiologic role. The twin data thus suggest that both genetic and environmental factors are significant in causing deafness.

Looking at twins, using audiometry to sharpen the diagnostic criteria, gives further information (Table IV). When a loss of 30

TABLE IV

STUDIES OF HEARING LOSS IN TWIN PAIRS
WHERE AT LEAST ONE TWIN IS DEAF (SANK, 1963)

Type of Twins	Complete Concordance	Concordance Using Threshold of > 30 db Loss	Complete Discordance	% Concordance at > 30 db Threshold
Monozygotic	10	5	2	88
Dizygotic	4	3	13	35
Total	14	8	15	

db A.S.A. or more is used as the criterion of concordance for deafness, the concordance for deafness is raised to 88 percent, approaching the theoretical 100 percent that would be present if the deafness were entirely genetic. This is a concordance increase of 29 percent in the identical twins as compared with a 16 percent increase in fraternal twins. These data suggest that less severe hearing losses are of the same genetic and environmental etiology as profound deafness and may be of prognostic value in genetic evaluation of families with deafness, as well as in developing genetic hypotheses about deafness.

The relatively high concordance of fraternal twins for childhood deafness may be the result of special factors related to twin pregnancies. In particular, the increased risk for prematurity in twins which is associated with an increased risk of deafness may result in a larger concordance between fraternal twins than might be expected among other types of siblings in which the gestation time and maternal disease history is not so highly correlated.

The Genetic Significances of Consanguinity

An excess of consanguinity, i.e., marriage of parents with recent common ancestors (cousins, uncle-niece, etc.), has genetic significance (Table II) in the greatly increased chance that two parents who have a recent common ancestor will each have the same recessive gene inherited from that common ancestor. Each could give a child this gene so that it would possess two such genes and be homozygous. Some genes in the homozygous state produce such recessive hereditary traits as childhood deafness. If the parents are first cousins and are normal, their children have at each locus one chance in sixteen of receiving from each parent a gene identical in origin that originally was carried in the heterozygous state by one of the common grandparents. This is in contrast to the small chance of a locus being homozygous in a child of a mating between genetically unrelated parents. Thus, if a gene has a frequency in the population of .001 (one per thousand), the chance of a marriage of first cousins producing a homozygote child is 63 per million, or 63 times the chance that two unrelated parents would produce such a homozygote. Since the possibility of a homozygote occurring by chance decreases with the square of the gene frequency, a gene with a frequency of .00001 (1 per 100,000) has more than 6,000 times the risk of occurring from a marriage of first cousins than from genetically unrelated persons. Conversely, the rarer a recessive gene, the more frequently will the parents of recessive homozygotes be related. This fact may be used to estimate the frequency of a rare recessive gene (Morton, 1962).

The Characteristics of Simply Inherited Traits

The definitive characteristics of simple hereditary traits are their patterns of transmission through families from generation to generation and their expected numerical frequencies among the children of parents who have known genetic constitutions. The genetic rules for these expectations are the basis for the distribution of hereditary deaf and normal children in family data. The genetic study of the distribution of deaf and normal children in families of various mating types is called segregation analysis (Morton, 1962).

The four simple modes of inheritance are autosomal dominant, autosomal recessive, sex-linked dominant, and sex-linked recessive. In autosomal dominant inheritance the trait results from the presence of at least one gene, of the possible two, of a particular type at a locus of a pair of autosomal chromosomes. The pattern of transmission of the trait in pedigrees is directly from parent to child, with every affected individual having an affected parent.

The exceptions to this rule are mutation and lack of expression. In mutation the gene is changed between the time it expresses itself in the parent and the time it appears in the child. Lack of expression, also called lack of penetrance, is the failure of an individual possessing the genetic structure that would be expected to result in the trait to demonstrate the trait. Mutation tends to increase the number of affected individuals detected, but it is a rare event. The expression of a genetic trait may vary from complete to nearly zero. It is theoretically independent of the mode of inheritance itself so that, in the case of dominantly inherited traits, it takes only one gene of an allelic pair to produce the trait in a given individual, and the penetrance measures the proportion of individuals with that gene that actually have the trait.

The expected proportion of children receiving a gene from a heterozygote parent is $1/2$ (Table V). In the case of rare dominant genes, usually only one parent has the gene, and that parent has only one such gene at a given locus and is, therefore, called a heterozygote. It is possible that a parent with the trait could have two genes producing the trait, one on each member of a chromosome pair, and thus be homozygous; but for rare traits this is much less frequent than the heterozygous state. If one parent has the trait and is a heterozygote, then he has one normal and one abnormal gene. Since he can pass only one of a gene pair to each child, each child has an equal chance of getting the normal or the abnormal gene, and the children of such a family will be, on the average, half affected heterozygotes and half normal. It is important to recognize that these are only theoretical expectations that cannot be applied rigidly to specific individual families where large chance deviations may occur, but only to large collections of families of a given genetic constitution.

In autosomal recessive inheritance the presence of the trait requires that both chromosomes of a given autosome pair have the same gene at the locus in question. The recessive nature of the trait is a result of the ability of one normal gene to do the job required for normal development and function. Thus the trait appears only when both genes on an autosome pair are of the abnormal type. The heterozygote individual, although having one normal and one abnormal gene, functions normally but is capable of passing the defective gene to his offspring.

TABLE V

THE THEORETICAL POSSIBILITIES OF SIMPLE INHERITANCE OF CHILDHOOD DEAFNESS WHERE D_i IS A DOMINANT GENE AT THE ith LOCUS PRODUCING DEAFNESS IN THE HETEROZYGOTE ($D_i d_i$) OR HOMOZYGOTE ($D_i D_i$) AND h_k IS A RECESSIVE GENE AT THE kth LOCUS GIVING DEAFNESS IN THE HOMOZYGOTE ($h_k h_k$)

Individuals are assumed to be homozygous normal at all loci not described.

Possible Genotypes and the Segregation Expected in Their Offspring

Phenotype of Mating	Genotype	Expected Deaf Offspring	Genotype	Expected Deaf Offspring	Genotype	Expected Deaf Offspring
Unaffected × Unaffected (U × U) or Acquired Deaf × Unaffected (AD × U)	$d_i d_i \times d_i d_i$ $d_i d_i \times d_j d_j$	0 0	$H_k H_k \times H_k H_k$ $H_p H_p \times H_k H_k$ $H_k h_k \times H_k H_k$ $H_k h_k \times H_p h_p$	0 0 0 0	$H_k h_k \times H_k h_k$ $H_p h_p \times H_p h_p$	¼ ¼
Hereditary Deaf × Unaffected (HD × U) or Hereditary Deaf × Acquired Deaf (HD × AD)	$D_i d_i \times d_i d_i$ $D_i D_i \times d_i d_i$	½ 1	$h_k h_k \times H_k H_k$ $h_k h_k \times H_p h_p$	0 0	$h_k h_k \times H_k h_k$	½
Hereditary Deaf × Hereditary Deaf (HD × HD)	$D_i d_i \times D_i d_j$ $D_i d_i \times D_j d_j$ $D_i D_i \times D_j d_j$ $D_i D_i \times h_k h_k$ $D_i d_i \times h_k h_k$	¾ ¾ 1 1 ½	$h_k h_k \times h_p h_p$	0	$h_k h_k \times h_k h_k$ $h_p h_p \times h_p h_p$	1 1

The pattern of recessive inheritance in pedigrees shows a clustering of affected individuals among brothers and sisters in sibships, the parents usually being normal functioning heterozygotes. There is an increased frequency of cousin marriages among the normal parents because of the effect this has of increasing the chance that hidden recessive genes from the common ancestors will come together in homozygous state in the offspring of parents with ancestors in common. When there are several sibships with affected children in a pedigree, there are frequently no affected individuals for several generations between them, so that the trait is said to "skip" generations.

Within sibships resulting from the mating of two recessive heterozygotes who have the potential for producing an affected homozygous offspring, the chance of any given fertilization being a homozygote is one of four (Table V). Thus when a sibship is identified as being of this mating type, one fourth of all children are expected to be affected.

It is of course not possible to identify such families in the general population until they have produced affected children. This results in a bias of considerable size, particularly if families are small. For example, if two heterozygotes produce only one child, in three fourths of these families the child will be normal and in one fourth affected. Three fourths of the couples who have only one child and who are capable of producing a recessive hereditary deaf child will not do so. The hearing child produced by this three fourths of the potential parents will, however be a carrier of the defective gene two thirds of the time. In two-child families of heterozygote parents, more than half will contain only hearing children, while only one child will be affected in six times as many families as those in which two children will be affected, so that the isolated deaf child with a hearing sibling is the usual situation in recessive hereditary deafness. Similarly, for three-child families more than 42 percent will escape having any affected children, and another 42 percent will have only one affected child. For four-child families 32 percent will not have any affected children and 42 percent will have only one affected child. These percentages demonstrate how the bulk of the recessive genes are present in the heterozygous and unexpressed condition.

In sex-linked traits, the genes are located on the X chromosome, of which females have two but which in the male is paired with the Y chromosome, which does not have any function in most traits. This has the effect of letting all genes present on the X chromosome in the male express themselves, while in the female the dominance relations act differently because in some cells the other X is functioning. Usually these effects are relatively slight compared with the over-all gene dominance effect.

The pedigree pattern of a sex-linked dominant is transmission of the trait without skips. Fathers only pass their X chromosomes to daughters. This pattern of father-daughter alternation is characteristic because affected fathers have only one X chromosome, so they must pass the gene to all their daughters and to none of their sons, who get the father's Y chromosome. Mothers, having two X chromosomes, may be heterozygotic for sex-linked traits.

In the dominant case for sex-linkage the trait is distributed equally between the sexes of the children of affected mothers, and half of each sex is affected. Affected fathers, in contrast, have all affected daughters and no affected sons. This assumes that the spouses of the affected heterozygotes are recessive homozygotes.

Sex-linked recessive traits have the striking characteristic that males, having one X chromosome, always show the trait if they have the gene predisposing to it, while females only show the trait in the homozygous state. This means that for a random-breeding population the frequency of affected females is the square of the frequency of affected males. For example, if .01 of males are deaf because of a sex-linked recessive gene, then .0001 of females would be expected to be homozygotes for that same gene and, therefore, also deaf. This ratio is 100 affected males for every affected female, and if the gene frequency decreases, the ratio of affected males to affected females increases.

In pedigrees, rare sex-linked recessive traits usually appear only in males or in daughters of affected fathers who have married a related female who is a heterozygote carrier. There is often increased consanguinity in these families.

Within the families of two normal parents where the female is a heterozygote for a sex-linked recessive trait, the expectation is that half of the sons will have the trait while half the daughters will appear normal, but will be heterozygous "carriers."

Although the genetic rules describing the expectation of the proportion of each genetic type of children from matings are discrete (Table V), for any particular human family it is nearly impossible to determine the genetic makeup of the parents and children. This is because the chances of particular combinations of children are not mutually exclusive. For example, in the case of a hereditary deaf person married to a normal person, it is possible that the deaf parent might be deaf because of a dominant gene in heterozygous condition or in homozygous condition. If this couple produces two deaf children, it is not possible to say which is the case. If, however, such a couple produces one deaf and one hearing child, the deaf parent must be a heterozygote. Similar reasoning may be applied to recessive pedigrees if enough information is available.

Unfortunately, most human sibships are small, and the exact knowledge of pedigree in modern society, particularly in America, is limited. This means that any one family does not contribute much information and, of course, all the different genetic mechanisms may be occurring together in a population from which data is collected.

The genetic analysis of such family data in which a character appears in some individuals is called segregation analysis, because it studies the way in which the character or trait segregates among the offspring of various types of matings (Morton, 1962). When sufficiently large bodies of data are available, these methods may be employed to estimate the types of genetic mechanisms that are acting and the proportional contribution of each type to the total. These methods, and their application to large bodies of data, are ideally suited to modern computer techniques.

Computer programs (SEGRAN) using maximum likelihood statistics have been applied by Dr. C. S. Chung (1960, 1964) to the segregation of deafness in Northern Ireland. The same methods will be applied by Dr. Chung to the data from Clarke School. The analysis presented here is based on his analysis of North Ireland data and on preliminary, less efficient hand calculations of the data from Clarke School and New York State (Table VI).

Population Genetics of Childhood Deafness

Among the modern population studies of deafness, some of which are quite large, (Furosho, 1957; Kittel and Schmoll-Esku-

TABLE VI

A COMPARISON OF THE OVER-ALL DISTRIBUTION OF CASES OF CHILDHOOD DEAFNESS CLASSIFIED BY PARENTAL MATING TYPE IN THREE POPULATION STUDIES

	North Ireland[a]		New York[b]		Clarke School[c]	
	Number	Percent	Number	Percent	Number	Percent
Acquired (usually both parents unaffected)	185	31.8	280	28.9	254	20.8
Unaffected × Unaffected (U × U), one child affected	219	37.7	501	51.7	521	42.6
Unaffected × Unaffected (U × U), more than one child affected	89	15.3	95	9.8	106	8.7
Hereditary Deaf × Unaffected (HD × U)	12	2.0	6[d]	.6	68	5.6
Acquired Deaf × Unaffected (AD × U)	1	.0			45	3.7
Hereditary Deaf × Hereditary Deaf (HD × HD)	48	8.3	86	8.9	143	11.7
Hereditary Deaf × Acquired Deaf (HD × AD)	26	4.5			71	5.8
Acquired Deaf × Acquired Deaf (AD × AD)	0				14	.1
Total	580		968		1,222	

a. From Stevenson and Cheeseman (1956).
b. From Sank (1963).
c. From Brown and Chung (1966).
d. By subtraction.

che, 1963; Lumio and Paljakka, 1964) only three done specifically for genetic objectives provide adequate data for segregation analysis. The large study of English deaf school children by Frazer (1964) has not been reported indetail but will undoubtedly be a major contribution to this area. Preliminary reports from this study will also be discussed here.

Stevenson and Cheeseman (1956) examined all the "deaf mutes" in Northern Ireland. This is a total ascertainment of a population of a limited size. It is analytically ideal but gives problems of interpretation because a small discrete population may not be genetically comparable with other populations.

The study of the New York State deaf population, as analysed by Sank (1963), is drawn from a large deaf population of more than 8,000. The analysis is however actually based on questionnaires completed by 688 adult deaf respondents who may not have been able to give accurate data on their relatives, or even on their own medical histories.

The Clarke School for the Deaf has collected pedigrees from parents of entering students for more than three decades (Hopkins, 1946). These records of 1,222 deaf children are the basis for the current efforts of the Human Genetics Branch of the National Institute of Dental Research. The records have been supplemented by interviews and physical examinations of a sample of the deaf students, alumni, and their parents and siblings. However, it has not been possible to compare Clarke pupils to the childhood deaf in general. It is clear that there is a larger portion of hereditary deaf attending Clarke than present in either the N. Ireland or New York State populations, but other differences, if any, appear genetically insignificant (Table VI).

The examination of the sex ratio among the childhood deaf shows (Table VII) that there is a significant excess of male deaf. This excess is most noticeable in the acquired group, which is defined as those in whom a prenatal or postnatal environmental factor has been claimed as a cause of deafness.

In the hereditary deaf group there is, at most, a very slight excess of males. This excess might be due to the failure to diagnose those diseases to which males are apparently more susceptible, with the resultant inclusion of these cases among the hereditary deaf, or it may be due to the presence of rare sex-linked genes. Some family pedigrees of deafness have been published which are very convincing as demonstrations of the expected pat-

TABLE VII

SEX RATIO OF CHILDHOOD DEAF IN SEVERAL POPULATIONS

Ref.	Studies	Number	Hereditary	Acquired	Total
25	N. Ireland[b]	424	.513		
12	Japan[c]	1,561	.502		
10	England[d]	2,355	.517	.578	.544
4	Clarke School	1,222	.512	.544	.519
15	Germany	2,788	.532[a]	.606	.567

a. Includes all cases diagnosed before 1 year of age.

b. From Stevenson and Cheeseman (1956).

c. From Furusho (1957).

d. From Fraser (1964), Brown and Chung (1964), Kittel and Schmoll-Eskuche (1963).

terns of sex-linked inheritance (Fraser, 1965), but it must be recognized that chance mimics of sex-linked patterns can occur in particular pedigrees of autosomal inheritance. Because of the very high sex ratio differential expected for rare sex-linked recessive traits, any appreciable gene frequency of sex-linked deafness would show itself by a marked excess of males. We may thus conclude that sex-linked genes, at one or many loci, do not contribute more than 2 percent of the hereditary childhood deafness in these three populations.

The frequency of consanguinity among normal hearing parents of the deaf is much greater than that present in the general population (Table VIII). In fact, it is much greater than would be pre-

TABLE VIII

THE FREQUENCY OF CONSANGUINEOUS MARRIAGES OF ALL

TYPES AMONG UNAFFECTED PARENTS OF THE DEAF (U × U) IN

THREE STUDIES COMPARED WITH POPULATION DATA

	N. Ireland[a]	New York[b]	Clarke School[c]
Total Consanguinity	.117	.121	.054
Population Estimate	.006	.001	

a. From Stevenson and Cheeseman (1956).

b. From Sank (1963).

c. From Brown and Chung (1966).

dicted on the basis of the observed frequency of deafness. This excess of consanguinity has been used by Chung (1959) to estimate the minimum number of recessive genes that might account for the observation. This estimation requires the assumption that all the recessive loci are equally frequent. Since this is probably not so, the values obtained must be considered to be only very rough estimates of the smallest number of genes. The deviation from this assumption will tend to make the estimate much smaller than the real case.

Estimation of a number of genes from consanguinity ratios requires a reliable estimate of the frequency of cousin marriages in the general population, which is not really available. It requires the assumption that the frequency of the trait in the general population be accurately known and uniform for the various groups from which all the consanguineous matings are derived. Because of the need to make these assumptions, the reliability of such estimates has been questioned (Neel, et al., 1963).

Despite the shaky assumptions, the method of consanguinity ratios gives similar estimates of between 30 and 150 recessive genes as the minimum number that might account for the observed consanguinity in these three populations. This result is supported by the result of an independent estimation method developed by Steinberg (1962) based on the frequency of affected cousins of the Clarke School probands which gives a preliminary estimate of about 80 genes.

As discussed above, it would be expected that among the deaf offspring of consanguineous matings a higher proportion would be deaf resulting from genetic factors than among the deaf offspring of normal parents in the general population (U x U). Thus consanguineous matings of U x U type provide an important test of the segregation ratio for deafness. If recessive genes play a major role, the segregation ratio in these matings should approximate .25.

Table IX shows that there is a shortage of deaf siblings of deaf probands in the total U x U matings from the expected .25 in all three populations. This shortage can be accounted for by supposing that the simple recessive genetic cases are diluted by a proportion of nongenetic cases or genetic cases which have segregation rates very much lower than .25. The validity of this hypothesis is supported by the segregation ratio in the consanguineous families, which does not differ from .25. It is

TABLE IX

SEGREGATION RATIOS OBSERVED IN U $\times$ U MATINGS

	N. Ireland[a]	New York[b]	Clarke School[c]
Total	.179 ± .012	.150 ± .010	.239 ± .008
Among Consanguineous	.269 ± .038	.250 ± .048	.244 ± .036
Among Relatives			.243 ± .025
U $\times$ U with Probands (adjusted)			.245 ± .017

a. From Stevenson and Cheeseman (1956).
b. From Sank (1963).
c. From Brown and Chung (1966).

further supported by the segregation ratios in families of relatives of Clarke School (U x U) probands and among all Clarke proband containing U x U families who have deaf relatives.

The good degree of fit of the segregation ratios strongly supports the hypothesis that among 75 percent of the families in which both parents are hearing, there is no history of significant illness in the deaf child, and there is no evidence of dominant inheritance of deafness in the pedigree, the deafness of the child may be attributed to simple autosomal recessive genes. Genetic or nongenetic nonsegregating factors are involved in about 25 percent of the families.

It must be stressed that these results are based on averages of a large number of families and do not prevent a small proportion of a balanced pattern of two other segregation ratios such as $1/2$ and $1/16$ from being included. There is no evidence, however, that this is occurring.

We thus conclude that about 25 percent of the families with two normal parents (U x U) in which only one child is deaf have no significant genetic potential for other deaf children, while among the remainder the genes causing deafness are segregating in a simple mendelian recessive pattern, so $1/4$ of all succeeding children might be expected to be deaf.

The marriages of two hereditary deaf (HD x HD) give more information about the genetics of deafness than any other class of matings (Table X), since several possible genotypes of parents can exist in this group. The matings of two recessive deaf, either give all-hearing offspring or all-deaf offspring, depending on whether the two parents are deaf from different or the same

TABLE X

OFFSPRING OF FERTILE HD × HD MATINGS IN THREE POPULATIONS

Type of Offspring	N. Ireland[a] Number	%	New York[b] Number	%	Clarke School[c] Number	%
All Hearing	21	65	57	79	84	64
All Deaf	5	16	7	10	33	25
Both Hearing and Deaf	6	19	8	11	15	11
Total	32		72		132	

a. From Stevenson and Cheeseman (1956).
b. From Sank (1963).
c. From Brown and Chung (1966).

TABLE XI

THE CONTRIBUTION OF DIFFERENT MODES OF INHERITANCE OF
THE HEREDITARY DEAF POPULATION AS ESTIMATED FROM THE
OFFSPRING OF HD × HD MATINGS IN TWO POPULATION GROUPS

Mating Type		N. Ireland[a]	Clarke School[b]
Recessive at Different Loci	h	.584 ± .108	.593 ± .004
Recessive at the same locus	y		.152 ± .027
Dominant	d	.223 ± .029	.255 ± .003

a. From Chung, et al. (1959).
b. From Brown and Chung (1966).

recessive genes (Table V). If one parent is deaf from heterozygous dominant genes, half of the offspring are expected to be
deaf; while if both are deaf from dominant heterozygous genes,
three fourths are expected to be deaf.

TABLE XII

THE APPROXIMATE CONTRIBUTIONS OF DIFFERENT ETIOLOGIC
FACTORS TO CHILDHOOD DEAFNESS IN THE UNITED STATES

25% Assignable extrinsic factors (Prenatal and Postnatal disease, trauma, etc.)

18% Non-segregating, unrecognized factors (Undiagnosed illness, poly-genes, etc.)

15% Autosomal dominant genes with penetrance of 80 to 100%

40% Autosomal recessive genes with 100% penetrance

< 2% Sex linked genes or other segregating genes with sex influence

Analysis shows (Table XI) about 15 percent of the matings of two hereditary deaf are between parents who are deaf from the same recessive genes and four fifths or 60 percent are between parents deaf from two different recessive genes. The matings of parents deaf from dominant genes contribute about 25 percent of the total and are somewhat more frequent in New York and Clarke than in North Ireland data.

Dominant genes producing childhood deafness in HD x HD matings have a penetrance, or frequency of expression, averaging between 80 and 100 percent. This is confirmed by study of the matings of the hereditary deaf with normal spouses (HD x U). The estimate of high penetrance of dominant genes is in agreement between the analyses of the North Ireland data (Chung, et al., 1959) and the Clarke School data (Brown and Chung, 1966). Sank (1963) arrived at a penetrance estimate of about 50 percent, which is significantly different from the other two. It appears likely that the difference reflects inadequate data about the hearing status of relatives provided by the deaf respondents in the New York State questionnaire study.

Thus, the observed pattern of offspring resulting from the marriages of two hereditary deaf is that 60 percent of the families contain only hearing children who are heterozygotes for two different recessive genes causing deafness but who are not deaf. Fifteen percent of the marriages of the hereditary deaf result in all-deaf children, since both parents are deaf from the same recessive genes and pass them to their children who are necessarily also homozygous and deaf. Another rare possibility that results in all-deaf children and may be included above is one parent homozygous deaf from a dominant gene. In 25 percent of the marriages of the deaf, one parent is deaf from a dominant gene in the heterozygous condition and passes this gene to half the children, but the remaining children are of normal hearing, although all the children are carriers of the recessive gene from the other parent who is presumably a recessive deaf.

The population and segregation analyses lead to the following conclusions (Table XII) regarding the frequency of factors causing childhood deafness: 25 percent result from assignable extrinsic factors; 18 percent from nonsegregating factors that may be complex genetic mechanisms or undiagnosed environmental factors, 15 percent from autosomal dominant genes with average penetrance of 80 to 100 percent; 40 percent from autosomal recessive genes at many loci with 100 percent penetrance; less than 2 percent sex-linked genes or other segregating genes with sex influence.

The 18 percent of families in which there is no assignable disease producing deafness, and in which there is no segregation, or at least segregation very much less than the expected $1/2$ or $1/4$ ratios, may represent undiagnosed disease of the types already identified as causing deafness or diseases yet unknown. These may also be cases of deafness from the cumulative effect of many genes acting together. Such polygenic inheritance does play a role in such traits as stature and body build and may also influence the development of normal hearing.

Genetic Implications of the Fitness of the Deaf

"The proportionate contribution of offspring to the next generation is called the *fitness* of an individual, or sometimes the *adaptive* value or selective value" (Falconer, 1960). If differences in fitness are related to the presence or absence of a particular gene or phenotype, then selection is said to be acting on the gene or phenotype. If individuals with a particular gene leave a smaller proportion of offspring than those with the other alleles at that particular locus, then the gene frequency in the following generation will decrease unless there is some compensation.

The deaf male in Northern Ireland has about one third the fitness of the hearing male (Stevenson and Cheeseman, 1956). This reduced fitness is due to both reduced frequency of marriage and to reduced fertility of the married deaf. In the Clarke data fitness is about three fourths of the value for hearing siblings for both sexes and is almost entirely a result of reduced fertility (Brown and Chung, 1966). The implication of these reductions in fitness is that in each generation there is a loss of the genes causing deafness. This should result in a steady decrease in the number of hereditary deaf. There is no evidence that this is the case. The question is thus raised, what is keeping the frequency of deafness at its present level?

There are two major mechanisms for maintaining a gene in a population in the face of selection against one of its phenotypes. A net mutation of the more advantageous gene to the less advantageous one can balance the loss resulting from selection. If one of the phenotypes containing the gene has a relative fitness advantage over all the other phenotypes, then this advantage may compensate the disadvantage of the other phenotype and maintain the gene in the population.

Application of the mutation theory to childhood deafness requires the assumption that the fitness of the deaf is and has been stable, and that the gene frequency has been stable for many generations. With these assumptions, using the estimated large numbers of recessive loci, we can calculate the mutation rates needed to balance the observed reduced fitness. These calculations result in average mutation rates of about 4×10^{-5} per locus for both the dominant and recessive loci using both the Irish data (Chung et al., 1959) and Clarke School data (Brown and Chung, 1966). Such mutation rates are well within the range that has been calculated for other human traits, so mutation alone would appear to be able to explain the presence of genetic childhood deafness.

The present evidence does not require that a selective advantage of any of the heterozygous forms of the recessive genes producing deafness be used to explain the frequencies observed. This does not deny the possibility that some of these genes may be maintained by some selective advantage in the heterozygote. The observations are quite compatible, however, with maintenance of genetic deafness in the population by mutation alone.

If mutation is the balancing source of the genes producing childhood deafness, this implies that there is a relatively constant base frequency of new genes that produce deafness appearing in each generation. At the present time there is no way of reducing this input of new genes. The selection against deafness by reduced reproductive fitness is the mechanism that keeps the frequency down in the population. As the education of the deaf and other social aspects related to occupational and economic opportunities for the deaf increase their fitness, it is to be expected that the frequency in the general population will increase somewhat.

When the population is mating at random in relation to the genes producing deafness, and these genes are individually very rare, it can be calculated that changes in the frequency of the gene will change the observed frequency of deafness in proportion to the ratio of the sums of the squares of the original and changed frequencies. Such a change will be proportionally greater for rarer genes. For genes as rare as one per hundred thousand, however, the change in frequency of deafness that would result from complete removal of the reduced fitness of the deaf is about 5 percent over a 10-generation period (Li, 1955). Nonrandom mating with respect to deafness certainly occurs and this would increase the change, but it would still not be very great.

The presence of many rare recessive genes in the general population implies that these are widely distributed in the heterozygous form among the apparently normal individuals. A rough estimate would suggest that about one fourth of the normal population carries at least one of the recessive genes causing deafness. Since there are many of these and each is rare, the chance of two randomly chosen individuals having the same gene is less than one in one thousand.

Childhood Deafness Associated with Syndromes

The association of childhood deafness with other defects has been repeatedly described (Fraser, 1964). There are more than fifteen named syndrome complexes of which deafness is apart (Lieber and Olbrich, 1959). Although these many associations have been known for years, it was not until recently that there has been any evidence about the relative frequency of these syndromes (Fraser, 1964; Brown and Chung, 1964). Most reports and syndrome descriptions are based on a limited number of cases. Frequently the deafness is not the primary interest of the investigator, so the recording of deafness in relatives is of variable reliability. Usually there is no audiologic or audiometric record. There is some possibility of confusion between mental deficiency and deafness in these descriptions.

In the multiple reports of some syndromes by different physicians, the descriptions of the syndromes are sufficiently variable to raise a question whether there are multiple forms of the same syndrome or whether there are actually several different syndromes, and whether the variations result from differences in genetic and environmental background or the presence of different major genes.

For example, Waardenburg, in the classic paper in which he first described the variations of the syndrome of dystopia canthis medialis lateroversa and associated congenital deafness (Waardenburg, 1951), recognized the variation present in the appearance of the individuals fitting his syndrome in the different families he reported but considered them to be genetically the same. In all families the pattern of inheritance is dominant with incomplete expression of the various components but the pattern of expression varies from family to family. Fisch (1959) pointed out a reasonable embryologic basis for the association of findings observed by Waardenburg and raised a reasonable doubt that the condition is a genetic entity. He suggested that it is a group of defects acting on a common developmental pathway. As yet there is no genetic test of these two hypotheses. Such a test would require collection of the data on offspring of marriages between two carriers of these genes, and, of course, these are so rare that the data would have to be collected from a variety of sources.

The same type of problems about possible heterogeneity are present for many of the other syndromes associated with childhood deafness. The methods of testing these syndromes are presently available but their power is so low that the mass of data needed would be prohibitively great for any one syndrome. If several syndromes were to be studied simultaneously, the relative cost of each evaluation might be less.

TABLE XIII

THE APPROXIMATE DISTRIBUTION OF VARIOUS CAUSES OF PROFOUND CHILDHOOD DEAFNESS IN 2,355 ENGLISH SPECIAL SCHOOL CHILDREN[a]

30 %	Assignable postnatal disease or trauma	26 %	Autosomal recessive undifferentiated
10 %	Perinatal insult, trauma, jaundice and prematurity	7.5%	Autosomal recessive with Goiter
6 %	Prenatal disease including Rubella in utero	3 %	Autosomal recessive with Retinitis Pigmentosa
2.5%	Craniofacial syndromes affecting hearing	1 %	Autosomal recessive with ECG abnormality
48.5%	Total Acquired	37.5%	Total Autosomal Recessive
		10 %	Autosomal dominant undifferentiated
		2.5%	Autosomal dominant with pigment abnormality
		12.5%	Total Autosomal Dominant
		1.5%	Sex Linked

a. From Fraser (1964).

Among the English deaf children (Table XIII) 2.5 percent had craniofacial syndromes affecting hearing (Fraser, 1964). These children result from a variety of disturbances of development of the face, skull, and neck which interfere with the development of a normal functioning ear. Included in this group might be those children with multiple congenital malformations and mental deficiency from major chromosome defects such as 13-15 trisomy; however, the limited data available on the chromosomes of congenital deaf children with several different syndromes has not revealed any major defect (Fraser, 1964).

The most frequently seen syndrome with children's deafness is that of Pendred (Table XIII). The presence of goiter which develops during childhood with congenital profound deafness has been well described as an autosomal recessive trait. It occurs in 7.5 percent of the English Special School Children and in a slightly higher proportion of the students and alumni of Clarke School. This syndrome has been associated with a specific enzyme defect in many cases (Thould and Scowen, 1964), but has also been found to occur in the absence of this defect (Hollander, et al., 1964).

By use of the test for the enzyme defect it has been found that half of the nongoiterous deaf children of one school had an enzyme deficiency (Baschieri, et al., 1963). Similar results have been obtained at the Clarke School. This finding suggests that the association of thyroid metabolism defects and deafness may be more frequent than can be diagnosed using the classic criteria of the Pendred syndrome. This association may have far-reaching significance for the study of the etiologic mechanisms in the production of congenital deafness.

The association of congenital deafness with a developing retinitis pigmentosa is the second most frequent of the identifiable syndromes (Table XIII). It is also inherited as an autosomal recessive trait but has a clinical heterogeneity which suggests that it may not be a single genetic entity. Because of the variable development of the retinitis, it may be present in a somewhat greater frequency than the 3 percent observed in England.

Fraser has discovered that about 1 percent of the childhood deaf have an abnormality of the electrocardiogram with associated syncopal episodes and sudden death. This syndrome has been observed at Clarke School. It may be wrongly diagnosed as epileptic seizure, but the EEG is normal and the EKG is grossly abnormal. Clinically, these children do not have any stupor after the fainting episode. This syndrome is probably underdiagnosed and can be detected from a painless half-minute EKG. This trait also appears to be inherited as an autosomal recessive, but the data about it are quite limited.

The association of pigmentary abnormalities with congenital deafness is present in several syndromes. These represent a continuum from partial albinism (Mende's syndrome) to a white tuft of hair on the scalp, or even a small depigmented patch of iris without hair changes (Waardenburg's syndrome). Conversely, the degree of hearing loss associated with the depigmentation varies from profound congenital bilateral deafness to unilateral deafness or unilateral mild loss within the same family.

The syndromes within this complex are inherited in an autosomal dominant manner in most cases, although one family has been reported as a sex-linked recessive (Fraser, 1964). The dominant forms account for about 2.5 percent of the childhood deaf in England and are of similar frequency at the Clarke School. As discussed above, there is considerable variability in this complex which makes both genetic and physiological evaluation difficult.

At the present time about one third of all hereditary deafness is associated with some other trait such as thyroid abnormality, retinitis pigmentosa, or depigmentation. It is hoped that future study will allow further classification of the yet undifferentiated cases into groups which will represent meaningful biological entities. When this separation is made, a meaningful genetic and physiological study of these individual groups will be possible, and it may also be possible to identify the normal parents who run special risks of having such children prior to their conception and through therapy prevent the defective development.

Summary

The genetics of deafness in childhood is not known in detail. The prevalence is probably around one per thousand by the age of normal speech development, but an unknown variability from population to population probably occurs. Studies of populations in Northern Ireland and New York State, and among the students and alumni of the Clarke School for the Deaf, Northampton, Massachusetts, are in general agreement that about 25 percent of childhood deafness can be attributed to identifiable prenatal or postnatal disease or trauma; 18 percent results from undiagnosed disease or genetic factors that have little chance of recurring in children produced by a given pair of parents; 15 percent is produced by several simple autosomal dominant genes with average penetrance of 80 to 100 percent; 40 percent of the childhood deaf result from homozygosity for a simple autosomal recessive gene of which there are estimated to be at least 30; while less than 2 percent are the result of sex-linked or sex-influence genes.

Most hereditary childhood deafness is not associated with an identified syndrome. Thyroid metabolism defect with or without goiter is the most commonly associated trait and appears to result from a variety of thyroid metabolism deficiencies of the recessive type. Disturbances of pigment metabolism are the only syndromes yet associated with dominant childhood deafness.

References

Baschieri, L., et al. 1963. "Evaluation and Limitations of the Perchlorate Test in the Study of Thyroid Function." *J. Clin. Endocrinol. & Metab.*, **23**:786–791.

Beasley, W. C. 1940. "The General Problem of Deafness in the Population." *Laryngoscope*, **50**:856–906.

Brown, K. S., and C. S. Chung. 1964. "Genetic Studies of Deafness at the Clarke School for the Deaf, Northampton, Mass." In *Report of the Proceedings of the International Congress on Education of the Deaf.* U. S. Government Printing Offfice Document 106, Washington, D. C.

Brown, K. S., and C. S. Chung. 1966. "Causes of Deafness at the Clarke School for the Deaf." Unpublished data.

Chung, C. S. 1964. "Applications of Digital Computers in Human Genetics." *Methods of Info. in Med.*, **3**:67–72.

Chung, C. S., O. W. Robison, and N. E. Morton. 1959. "A Note on Deaf Mutism." *Ann. Hum. Genet.*, **23**:357–366.

Falconer, D. S. 1960. *Introduction to Quantitative Genetics*. New York: The Ronald Press Company.

Fisch, L. 1955. "Aetiology of Congenital Deafness and Audiometric Patterns." *J. Laryng. & Otol.*, **69**:479–493.

Fisch, L. 1959. "Deafness as Part of an Hereditary Syndrome." *J. Laryng. & Otol.*, **73**:355–382.

Fraser, G. R. 1964. "Profound Childhood Deafness." *J. Med. Genet.*, **1**:118–150.

Fraser, G. R. 1965. "Sex-Linked Recessive Congenital Deafness and the Excess of Males in Profound Childhood Deafness." *Ann. Human Genet.*, **29**:171–196.

Furusho, T. 1957. "A Genetic Study on the Congenital Deafness." *Jap. J. Human Genet.*, **2**:35–58.

Hollander, C. S., *et al.* 1964. "Congenital Deafness and Goiter." *Am. J. Med.*, **37**:630–637.

Hopkins, Louise A. 1946. "Studies on the Inheritance of Deafness in the Pupils of the Clarke School for the Deaf." *Laryngoscope*, **56**:570–601.

Kittel, G., and G. Schmoll-Eskuche. 1963. "Statistische Erhebungen zur Atiologie Ererbter und fruh Erworbener Hochgradiger Perzeptions-storungen." *Archiv. Ohren- usw. Heilk. u. Z. Hals- usw. Heilk.*, **181**:310–328.

Li, C. C. 1955. *Population Genetics.* The University of Chicago Press.

Lieber, B. and G. Olbrich. 1959. *Worterbuch der Klinischen Syndrome.* 2nd ed., Munchen-Berlin: Urban and Schwarzenberg.

Lumio, Jaakko S. and Pertti Paljakka. 1964. "Tutkimuksia Suomen Kuurojenkeskisista Aviolilitoista" (Studies on Marriages Between Deaf People in Finland). *Duodecim*, Suppl. XLIII.

Morton, N. E. 1962. "Segregation and Linkage." In Burdette, Walter J. (ed.), *Methodology in Human Genetics.* San Francisco: Holdon-Day.

Neel, J. V., H. B. Hamilton, T. Y. Kobara and K. Ozaki. 1963. "The Uneven Distribution in Japan of Carriers in Rare Recessive Gene Causing Acatalasemia and the Implications for Studies on Inbreeding Effects." In Goldschmidt, E. (ed.). *The Genetics of Migrant and Isolate Populations.* Williams and Wilkins.

Powers, Margaret H. 1964. Bureau of Physically Handicapped Children. Board of Education, Chicago (Presented at Conference on Collection of Health Statistics of Severe Hearing Impairments and Deafness in the U. S.).

Sank, Diane. 1963. "Genetic Aspects of Early Total Deafness." In Rainer, J. D. (ed.). *Family and Mental Health Problems in a Deaf Population.* New York: Columbia University.

Santillan, J. S., *et al.* 1965. "Hereditary Deafness; Two Distinct Pedigrees and Ways of Rehabilitation." *J. Philipp. Med. Assoc.*, **41**:475–482.

Steinberg, A. G. 1962. "Population Genetics: Special Cases." In Burdette, Walter J. (ed.), *Methodology in Human Genetics.* San Francisco: Holdon-Day.

Stevenson, A. C., and E. A. Cheeseman. 1956. "Hereditary Deaf Mutism, with Special Reference to Northern Ireland." *Ann. Hum. Genet.*, **20**:177–207.

Thould, A. K., and E. F. Scowen. 1964. "The Syndrome of Congenital Deafness and Simple Goiter." *J. Endocrin.*, **30**:69–77.

Waardenburg, P. J. 1951. "A New Syndrome Combining Developmental Anomalies of Eyelid, Eyebrows and Nose Root with Pigmentary Defects of Iris and Head Hair with Congenital Deafness." *Am. J. Human Genet.*, **3**:195–253.

SURGICAL TREATMENT OF HEARING LOSSES IN CHILDREN

CONDUCTIVE-TYPE hearing losses are a common finding in children. Some of these losses are amenable to correction while others are not, depending on the degree of alteration of structure or anomaly underlying the hearing loss. Differential diagnosis and therapy are based on an accurate history and careful physical and audiological examinations. The various conditions and their relation to each other which result in a conductive hearing loss and the possible surgical treatment will be discussed.

Retention of Fluid in the Middle-Ear Space (Secretory Otitis Media)

This phenomenon known as middle-ear effusion is a common and frequent cause for prolonged mild but important conductive losses in children. Its recognition is important, not only because of the associated hearing handicap, but it may be the forerunner of serious chronic alterations in the middle ear and mastoid if not corrected. This condition may be the first stage in the development of a cholesteatoma, the differential in atmospheric and middle-ear pressure present resulting in an invagination of squamous epithelium which invades the middle ear and mastoid process. Lesser changes in structure, such as retraction pockets in the middle ear, may result in absorption of portions of the ossicular chain and adhesive processes involving the ossicular chain, oval and round windows, and, in some instances, the whole extent of the middle ear. The basis for the development and maintenance of the fluid is usually faulty ventilation of the middle ear through the eustachian tube as a result of alteration of the physiology of the upper respiratory tract. Such alterations result from abnormalities of development of the eustachian tube, with associated poor development of the palate (varying in degrees from bifid uvula and short palate to gross abnormalities, such as cleft palate) and allergic and infectious processes which involve the structures of the nasopharynx and nasal fossae and related sinuses. These factors are often combined in various degrees.

The fluid retained in the middle ear may be of serous or mucoid character, depending upon the degree of associated infection which is common and the nature of the reaction in the middle-ear mucosa. In the presence of long-standing retention of fluid, the mucosa of the middle ear undergoes definite changes, the fluid becomes mucoid and viscid, and the ear has been described as a "glue ear," since the retained material resembles glue in this chronic stage.

While the treatment of this condition is not entirely surgical, this type of intervention may aid in correction of the condition in selected cases. A common underlying cause for retention of fluid in the middle ear is nasal allergy. Other associated conditions are bacterial infection in the ethmoid and maxillary sinuses and hypertrophy and infection in the adenoid. All of these conditions may result in lymphatic stasis in the region of the eustachian tube with resulting edema and alteration of the physiology of the eustachian tube and middle-ear mucosa. In former years, the condition was thought to be entirely surgical with adenoidectomy and paracentesis of the tympanic membrane the treatment of choice. With the development of an appreciation for allergy of the upper respiratory tract as a basis for disturbed physiology, however, it is now known that nasal allergy and its frequent associated complication of sinusitis, particularly involving the ethmoid, can in itself be the underlying cause for subacute and chronic fluid in the ear or "secretory otitis media." Respiratory allergy and sinusitis must therefore be ruled out by thorough history and physical examination before surgical intervention, especially if adenoidectomy is considered. Once the diagnosis of nasal allergy is established, appropriate allergic therapy is indicated. Paracentesis and ventilation of the middle-ear space by temporarily placing a small plastic ventilating tube through the tympanic membrane may be necessary for improvement in·

hearing. Treatment of the allergic condition by hyposensitization measures and of the infection by specific antibiotics may be necessary over an extended period before the altered state of the upper respiratory tract is restored to normal function with resulting ventilation of the middle-ear space and improvement in hearing.

In some of these patients, adenoidectomy is required, but this should not be considered until nasal allergy and sinusitis have been ruled out, since it is well known that the adenoidectomy alone is not effective in the presence of these two other common associated causes for eustachian-tube dysfunction. Exacerbations of purulent acute otitis media are common in the presence of subacute and chronic secretory otitis media. Recurrent severe otalgia, rupture of the tympanic membrane, and purulent ear drainage are the associated signs and symptoms. When the underlying basis for the problem is unrecognized and the acute suppurative infection is treated by antibiotics alone, the acute suppurative phase of the ear infection is controlled, and the chronic phase of the secretory condition remains. As long as the basis for the condition is unrecognized or ignored and untreated, a vicious cycle may exist, leading to chronic complications and conductive hearing loss.

Physical examination of the tympanic membrane in the presence of eustachian tube dysfunction and fluid retention in the middle ear reveals characteristic changes in light reflex, amber discoloration or other changes in color of the membrane, signs of retraction and, a change in contrast between the membrana tympani and the malleus, which are well known to the experienced examiner. When in doubt, paracentesis should be performed to confirm the diagnosis. Before the treatment is instituted, however, audiological tests with pure tone air conduction and bone conduction studies as a minimal requirement are indicated. The assumption that a pure conduction loss is present should not be made merely on the presence of retained fluid in the middle ear. The conductive loss caused by the fluid may be superimposed on a sensorineural loss. In the absence of appropriate pretreatment examination, many posttherapy disappointments may occur for parent and physician alike. When combined losses are present in association with fluid retention, however, therapy for the condition underlying the conductive loss is indicated. Since the combined loss is more profound under these conditions, and the patient is usually afflicted by recurrent acute ear infections, as the fluid ear is highly susceptible to bacterial invasion, the appropriate treatment should be promptly instituted.

Chronic Suppuration and Resulting Damage to the Sound-Conduction Mechanism

While the erroneous notion still persists in many quarters that antibiotic therapy will control all types of ear infections, acute and chronic, destructive lesions of the tympanic membrane (persistent tympanic perforation) and ossicular chain (absorption and erosion of the ossicles) are relatively common findings in the presence of or as a result of chronic suppuration of the middle ear. Cholesteatoma formation may be associated. It is true that antibiotic therapy effectively controls the large majority of acute infections of the middle ear, but necrotizing processes in relation to the tympanic membrane may have been so advanced before therapy is started that persistent perforation of the tympanic membrane is a sequela. Invasion of skin through the perforation or in an area of the membrane weakened by the infection, or a retraction pocket may develop in the presence of eustachian tube dysfunction, with the result that a cholesteatoma develops in the middle ear space and/or the mastoid antrum. Such persistent perforations, associated or not with cholesteatoma, are commonly associated with chronic suppuration and destruction of the conduction apparatus in the middle ear. If unilateral, the hearing impairment is not as handicapping, but whether unilateral or bilateral, the condition is one to cause concern for future health and hearing conservation. Suppuration and resulting ear drainage do not always occur in the presence of cholesteatoma, however, since cholesteatoma may develop from a retraction of a portion of the tympanic membrane alone. In such a case, conductive hearing loss may be the first symptom of the disease. The importance of a thorough physical examination cannot be overemphasized in the complete diagnosis of established and impending conductive hearing losses. Cholesteatoma and its underlying dangers to the general health and well being of the individual involved may be missed as the cause for conductive hearing loss in the absence of thorough physical examination by the specialized or expert examiner. Unfortunately, these subtle early changes in the tympanic membrane often are unrecognized and severe complications follow.

In the presence of chronic perforation of the tympanic membrane and other lesions of the conduction apparatus, the question arises whether surgical repair of such lesions (tympanoplasty) is possible and practical in childhood. In answer, it can be stated that provided certain basic requirements are met, the tympanoplastic repair of such lesions are possible. The objective of tympanoplasty is to control the disease in the temporal bone and to conserve or improve hearing by reconstructing the conduction mechanism (tympanic membrane and ossicular chain). The presence of associated cholesteatoma with retention of squamous debris usually demands surgical intervention.

Considering the possibility of repair of the tympanic perforation and ossicular chain, the underlying condition responsible for the destruction is considered before surgical therapy is contemplated. If the patient is an allergic individual and this underlying diathesis has been the basic cause for repeated acute ear infections and/or cholesteatoma, the basic cause for the ear problem must be brought under satisfactory control and such status maintained before successful tympanoplastic repair can be hoped for. This concept applies to patients of all ages. Thus, in children, tympanoplasty operations are possible if the proper preoperative criteria are met. If it is observed that upper respiratory infections and allergic symptoms persist, any such tympanoplastic operations are postponed until proper control of the allergic condition is realized. Eosinophilic granuloma which should be suspected by bilateral drainage from the ears, characteristic X-ray findings of marked destruction in the cellular elements of the temporal bone may be a cause of conductive loss which can be confused with chronic suppurative mastoiditis. Biopsy when properly performed establishes the diagnosis of eosinophilic granuloma, which is best treated with Chlorambucil.

Congenital Anomalies of the Ear

Various malformations of a congenital nature are recognized causes for unilateral and bilateral conductive hearing losses. Malformations of the external and middle ear, combined or separate, may occur with a resulting pure conduction loss but may also be associated with a congenital sensorineural loss of any degree. In patients with congenital deformity in the middle ear and with normal auditory canals and tympanic membranes, the history of hearing loss since birth is a characteristic finding as opposed to acquired abnormalities of the ossicular chain. In patients with sensorineural component, special attention in bone conduction testing is necessary in determining which patients have a true conductive component as opposed to those who have an apparent conductive element as a result of feeling the vibration of the bone conduction oscillator instead of hearing it. A pseudo-air bone gap is often found in young children with pure sensorineural losses as a result of the child's response to the bone conduction stimulation through feeling the vibration without being able to verbalize this sensation as older children and adults can. A word of caution is in order in this regard as well as in relation to the advisability for an attempt at surgical correction of the conductive element of established combined losses, especially when the bone-conduction findings can be recorded for only the lower three frequencies in the speech range. The reported results of such operations are equivocal and the problem deserves more detailed study before further attempts are considered.

Congenital Aplasia of the External Auditory Canal

The condition may be unilateral or bilateral and result in a partial or complete obstruction of the canal with varying degrees of conductive hearing loss up to an average loss of fifty decibels when complete obstruction is present. The anomaly results from abnormal development in the ossification centers in the tympanic plate with the possible result that the bony portion of the auditory canal is obstructed by dense bone, which may extend from the usual position of the tympanic membrane to the isthmus of the external auditory canal. The skin lining of the canal ends in a pit in the bone at this point, as a rule, but when the obstruction is not complete, an hour-glass effect may be present with skin lining the complete canal, which is narrowed at the isthmus. Squamous debris in profuse amounts may be found medial to the constriction when this type of deformity is present. The degree of obstruction may be determined by the judicious palpation with a small probe, X-ray and audiological examinations (Figure 1).

Associated deformities of the ossicular chain, especially of the malleus and incus, are common findings. The stapes may be congenitally fixed or deformed and the oval and round windows altered. The tympanic membrane is often replaced by a plate of

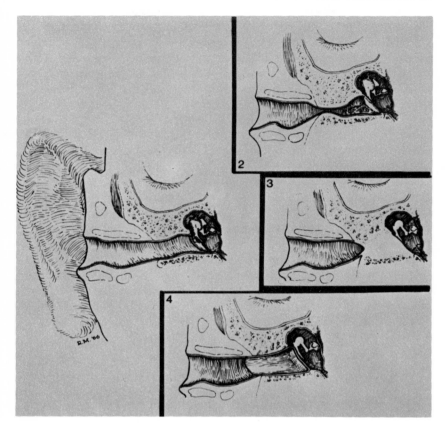

Figure 1. Various anomalies of the external auditory canal in #2 and #3 are compared with the normal canal in the main figure. Note the ossicular deformity in #3 commonly associated with congenital aplasia of the canal. In #4 the usual method for application of a skin graft to the ossicular chain following removal of the bony obstruction in the canal is illustrated.

bone, which may be the medial surface of the obstructing mass in the canal. The malleus is usually fused to this plate in an irregular manner, and varying degrees of deformity of the incus are seen. In some cases, however, the incus and stapes are practically normal in configuration.

Surgical correction of the condition should be considered cautiously. In unilateral cases with practical hearing in the uninvolved ear, surgery for improvement of hearing in the involved ear is not indicated. Before surgery is contemplated in bilateral cases, several factors should be considered. The anatomical deformity can be judged by the recognition of the facial symmetry, since facial deformity may be associated (Treacher-Collins syndrome), palpation to aid in determining the development of the mastoid, probing to determine the depth of the external auditory canal, and by detailed roentgenographic studies to determine the pneumatization and development of the temporal bone. Patients with hemiatrophy of the face usually have the least temporal-bone development on the side of the face exhibiting the atrophy. In the absence of atrophic changes in the face, the temporal bone pneumatization as shown by X-ray may be practically absent. In these patients with poor pneumatization, a middle-ear cleft may not be present, the facial nerve may be aberrant in course or deformed and thus more susceptible to injury. In the absence of an adequate middle ear cleft, surgical correcton is not feasible.

Other factors to be considered are the degree of hearing restoration possible and the postoperative care of the newly formed external canal. In the operation, the obstruction in the canal is removed with the cutting burr and the ossicular chain exposed. If the chain is mobile, a tympanic membrane and canal lining is formed by the application of a split-thickness skin-graft to the area, in contact with the incus and malleus remnant. When the stapes is fixed or the oval window not developed, a fenestration of the lateral semicircular canal is advised, provided the round window is present. Following this maneuver, a skin-graft may be applied to the fenestra and tympanic membrane and canal area. In these patients with normal bone conduction, the hearing is rarely improved to an average level of thirty-two decibels (ISO) and a forty-two decibel level is considered a good result. Postoperative care of the canal may be troublesome because the canal is irregular in shape, is lined with skin-containing appendages from the external surface of the body, and healing may be incomplete. For these reasons, this type of surgery should only be attempted by, or under the direct supervision of, a surgeon of wide experience in this field. Certainly a hearing aid is advised during the age of speech development and should be considered as the rehabilitative method of choice in many instances. Such a patient should be carefully considered before surgery is attempted.

*Middle-Ear Deformity in the Presence of Normal External
Auditory Canal*

Malformation of the ossicles in the presence of a normal pinna
and external auditory canal is fairly frequent but may be associated with other deformities of the face. In the presence of ossicular deformities, changes in the appearance of the tympanic
membrane may be evident on physical examination. Pure conductive losses of moderate to severe degree are common audiologic
findings in all of these ossicular deformities, the degree of loss
depending on the extent of the deformity (Figure 2):

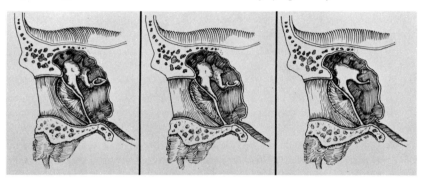

Figure 2. Various degrees of ossicular deformity, including congenital
fixation of the stapes as seen in the left-hand figure, abnormalities of the
footplate and oval window as seen in the middle figure, and abnormalities
of all ossicles and oval window as seen in the right-hand figure may be
present.

1. The malleus may be irregular in shape or position and may
be fused to the annulus posteriorly by a bar of bone. This
deformity usually can be recognized on examination of the tympanic membrane.

2. Deformity of the incus: While abnormal development involving the incus alone is not common, it has been encountered on occasion with fusion of the medial surface of the body
of the incus to the surface of the lateral semicircular canal by
a bar of bone. Such fixation is not to be confused with fixation of the incus from other causes, such as tympanosclerosis.

3. Congenital fixation or malformation of the stapes and oval
window: The stapes and oval window may be malformed in the
presence of normal malleus and incus. The most common mal-

formation is so-called congenital fixation of the stapes, which is really an abnormality of development of the otic capsule in the area of the oval window. The window is usually slightly smaller than the footplate, and the footplate edge is fused over the window as a lid rather than being suspended in the window by the annular ligament attachment.

All degrees of malformation in this area have been encountered, including complete absence of the stapes and oval window with the associated finding of the facial nerve coursing through the oval-window area or inferior to it. An interesting irregularity of development of the stapes has been encountered occasionally in the presence of pure conduction, as well as mixed losses, in that the stapes has been only partially formed with absent posterior crus and small round footplate attached to the anterior crus. Again, in these cases, the small footplate seemed to fit like a lid with a beveled edge on a small oval window.

4. Malformation of all ossicles: This deformity may occur independently of other deformities of the ear and also in conjunction with aplasia of the external auditory canal. The ossicles may be entirely irregular in shape, fused together, and immobile. Deformities of one or both windows may be so marked that the usual landmarks of the middle ear are not recognizable.

Surgical Treatment of Malformation of the Ossicles

In children with true conductive losses and the typical history as mentioned above, surgical exploration of the middle ear is indicated, provided the upper respiratory physiology is normal. All the possibilities of the abnormality should be conveyed to the parents before surgery. Fixation of the malleus or incus in the presence of a normal mobile stapes can be corrected and a mobile functioning chain re-established by removal of the fixating process and repositioning of the incus if necessary. Congenital fixation of the stapes may be a problem, in spite of the fact that stapedectomy and the use of a prosthesis in the oval window is a commonly performed successful operation in the adult. In our relatively small series of thirteen children with congenital fixation of the stapes, we have encountered four who exhibited free-flowing perilymph from the oval window coincident with stapedectomy in three patients and on an attempt at mobilization in one. Each of these three patients had an increased loss of hearing, on a sensorneural basis, following the operation. An increased incidence of abnormal circulation of labyrinthine fluids (presumed to be caused by an abnormally wide cochlear aqueduct) may be associated with congenital fixation of the stapes.

In patients having gross abnormalities of the oval window preventing surgical approach in this area, the fenestration operation in later adulthood is a possibility, if the round window is functional. The fenestration operation is rarely indicated in children because of the increased rate of bone metabolism in the growing child.

Otosclerotic Fixation of the Stapes

This condition is believed to be rare in children under the age of twelve but is a possibility to be considered. We have encountered two patients with proven otosclerosis at surgery who had a history of conductive loss since age ten years. The history of progressive conductive loss in the absence of other findings, such as fluid in the middle ear, inflammation or abnormality of the tympanic membrane, suggests otosclerosis as a possibility. Surgical exploration reveals the type and degree of the abnormality. In children with minor to moderate degrees of otosclerotic fixation, stapedial surgery in the form of partial or total stapedectomy may be performed. The two patients cited above have been successfully rehabilitated for three and five years respectively. Young adults with proven otosclerosis, however, occasionally have a fulminating type of otosclerotic lesion in the oval window. Considerable speculation has occurred regarding the advisability of surgery in young otosclerotics for this reason, since closure of the oval window by regrowth of otosclerotic bone may occur rather rapidly following surgery in the presence of the fulminating otosclerosis (markedly involved footplate). In our experience with this age group (24 patients), the patient with average degrees of otosclerotic involvement has received definite benefit from the surgery. The overall results in this age group, however, are not as good as those obtained in the older age groups. If the process is of the fulminating type, its characteristics may be suspected by the rapidity of the loss over this period and proved by exploratory operation. If the loss has been slowly progressive, the fulminating type is probably not present.

Summary

The importance of the normal physiology of the upper respiratory tract as related to middle-ear ventilation is evident in a discussion of conductive hearing losses in children, since allergic manifestations and upper-respiratory infection are commonly found in this age group. In subacute and chronic secretory otitis media, one or both of these conditions may be the underlying etiology and, in the presence of other causes for conductive losses, may be a complicating factor which alters the prognosis if uncontrolled. In those patients in this age group with adequate upper-respiratory function, surgical rehabilitation of hearing can be an effective method depending upon the degree of abnormality. In patients with irreversible changes in physiology and structure, amplification with a hearing aid is obviously the method of choice.

AUDITORY PATHWAY LESIONS
RESULTING FROM Rh INCOMPATIBILITY

ORTH (1875) described yellow pigment in the basal ganglia of the brain in newborn infants with jaundice. Schmorl (1904) coined the term "kernicterus" to designate jaundice of various cranial nuclear masses (or "grisea," as they are now termed). The term "kernicterus" later took on a clinical context, describing extrapyramidal spasticity with athetoid choreiform patterns, occasionally including varying degrees of mental retardation.

The primary cause of kernicterus was considered a congenital hemolytic disease, presumably resulting from fetal hematogenous sepsis; thus the term "septic jaundice of the newborn" was also used to describe what was later termed erythroblastosis fetalis, which was clinically a synonym for congenital hemolytic disease.

The entity of erythroblastosis fetalis occurred in infants who showed an abnormal retention of immature erythrocytes or erythroblasts in the neonatal blood stream. This condition was a serious disease and was frequently fatal. In its most severe form, the baby was born dead, and this variety of the lesion was termed congenital fetal hydrops. In a less severe form, a viable infant was born but was jaundiced at birth or became jaundiced within the first day of birth. This clinical entity was termed icterus gravis neonatorum, and it also carried a fairly high mor-

From the Head and Neck Surgery Division, Otology Section, University of California, Los Angeles, with grateful acknowledgment to the Hope for Hearing Research Foundation.

tality rate. If these infants survived, they would then frequently show clinical evidence of kernicterus and severe anemia. The least serious form of the disease occurred in the child born with no apparent abnormalities but who developed severe anemia, with or without mild or moderate jaundice, several days postnatally. This least serious version of erythroblastosis fetalis was termed congenital hemolytic anemia, and only occasionally did such children develop kernicteric sequelae.

The Rhesus Factor

When Landsteiner and Wiener (1940) first described a new agglutinogen for human erythrocytes, they termed it the "Rh factor" because a similar agglutinogen was found in the erythrocytes of the Rhesus monkey. All persons whose red cells lacked the Rh agglutinogen were considered "Rh negative," and those individuals whose cells possessed the Rh agglutinogen were termed "Rh positive." Rh negative individuals do not normally have anti-Rh agglutinins in their plasma, but Rh negative individuals are likely to form antibodies if Rh agglutinogen is introduced into the circulation in either of two ways. The most common cause is pregnancy when Rh agglutinogen from an Rh positive father crosses the placenta of an Rh negative woman pregnant with an Rh positive fetus, the fetus having inherited the Rh agglutinogen from the father. A less common cause is the introduction of Rh agglutinogen in Rh negative persons of both sexes when transfused with Rh positive blood.

The discovery of the Rh factor did away with the old conception of fetal hematogenous sepsis as the primary cause of erythroblastosis fetalis, and today the primary cause of erythroblastosis fetalis is considered to be the presence of Rh antibodies in the maternal blood of an Rh negative woman. An Rh negative woman whose Rh positive husband is homozygous for Rh can expect all of her children to be Rh positive. If her husband is heterozygous for Rh, an Rh negative woman can expect half of her children to be Rh positive. Thus, during pregnancy, the blood of an Rh positive fetus escapes from the placenta into the maternal circulation, and in an Rh negative mother, antibodies against these cells may be produced by the mother. These antibodies then pass from the maternal blood into the fetal circulation and destroy Rh positive cells of the fetus by combining with them, producing the end state of erythroblastosis fetalis.

Unless the mother has been previously transfused with Rh positive blood and has developed antibodies, or has had a previous pregnancy resulting in an abortion, a first-born child rarely will have erythroblastosis fetalis, since it is unusual to find sufficient concentration of antibodies during the course of a first pregnancy to harm the fetus. However, once the concentration of antibodies responsible for hemolytic disease in the newborn has been developed in the mother, subsequently conceived Rh positive fetuses may suffer from hemolytic disease as a result of the iso-immunization and the maternal antibodies that have persisted from the previous pregnancy. (It should be mentioned, of course, that in addition to the classic etiology on an Rh basis, ABO incompatibilities and other rare blood incompatibilities may also cause erythroblastosis fetalis.)

Any condition causing hemolysis, caused either by Rh or ABO incompatibility, can cause an accumulation of indirect bilirubin from hemoglobin breakdown, resulting in jaundice. Bilirubin is indirect bilirubin until conjugated enzymatically in the liver to direct bilirubin. In some infants, physiologic jaundice may occur because of a temporary insufficiency of the enzyme glucuronyl transferase. If bilirubin levels in the newborn exceed 12 mg.% in full term or 15 mg.% in premature infants, physiologic jaundice will result.

While hyperbilirubinemia is necessary for the development of kernicterus, it cannot be considered the sole factor. It appears that hypoxia of varying degrees may be a necessary prerequisite for the development of bilirubin deposition in cranial regions. Indirect bilirubin is lipid soluble and thus apparently has an unusual affinity for brain tissue. Most hematologists and pediatricians consider the crucial level of bilirubin concentration to be 20 mg.%. Any retention in excess of that figure usually will produce clinical sequelae. The blood-brain barrier permeability appears to be greater in prematures, and thus prematurity seems to be another factor predisposing to kernicterus.

Phelps (1941) and Coquet (1944) described the presence of a peculiar type of hearing loss in athetoid cerebral palsied children. In a paper discussing educational problems of congenital perceptive deafness in children (Goodhill, 1947) I stated,

Several congenitally deaf children of Rh negative mothers are now being studied. Subclinical erythroblastosis in the newborn may have etiological significance in some cases of congenital perceptive deafness. It is quite possible that changes similar to kernicterus occur in the cochlea or in the ascending auditory tracts.

In 1949, I reported a group of cases before the American Acad-, emy of Ophthalmology and Otolaryngology under the heading of "Nuclear Deafness" (Goodhill, 1950), which included children with varying varieties and degrees of sensorineural hypacusis and dysacusis. They all had in common a definite history of erythroblastosis fetalis due to Rh-factor incompatibility. The majority were athetoid spastics with deafness, but a few had no other neurologic sequelae.

Since it had been known for years that kernicterus may involve varying portions of the brain stem, including dorsal and ventral cochlear nuclei, and since a rather unusual bilateral symmetry of the threshold audiograms was revealed in the study of my cases, I suggested the term "nuclear deafness" to describe the auditory lesion. A study of three pairs of temporal bones from erythroblastotic newborns by Dr. Dorothy Wolff in 1956 showed an absence of end-organ involvement but demonstrated some cellular degeneration in the spiral cochlear ganglion, which I considered possibly to be secondary to cranial cochlear nuclear hyperbilirubinemic lesions. Since there were other manifestations of interference with communication in "aphasoid" and similar "dysacusic" lesions, probably caused by cortical or subcortical lesions, the Rh factor definitely seemed to be indicted as an etiologic factor in a special type of rather diffuse and varied "central deafness."

In these temporal bones, the spiral ganglion cells revealed vacuolar degenerative changes of their cytoplasm in all turns, characteristic of hypoxia, although the number of spiral ganglion cells appeared to be normal. These degenerative changes in the spiral ganglion cells were in marked contrast to normal-appearing vestibular ganglion cells. The nerve fibers in the bony spiral lamina appeared normal in number, the organ of Corti was present everywhere, and the hair cells were identifiable.

Crabtree and Gerrard (1950) reported 22 cases of kernicterus of which 18 were examined otologically, utilizing conventional otologic examinations and play audiometry. Their material showed audiometric patterns comparable to those reported in my 1949 report.

They were able to report examination of the brain stem and temporal bones of one neonate dying of erythroblastosis fetalis and severe generalized jaundice. They reported that both organs of Corti and auditory nerve fibers and ganglion cells were normal. Examination of the brain stem, however, showed marked changes in both ventral and dorsal cochlear nuclei. The cell bodies of the nerves were gone, and in some the cytoplasm was strangely similar to the pyramidal cell damage seen in hippocampus areas in typical kernicterus.

In analyzing their data, Crabtree and Gerrard noted very little relationship between the extent of the hearing loss and the degree of extrapyramidal damage, a finding quite similar to my observation, and they pointed out that bile stains had been discovered in the cochlear nerve nucleus in a case of kernicterus by Beneke (1907), Bertrand (1946) and Potter (1947). They thus concluded that in "deafness associated with kernicterus, the organs of hearing develop normally, but the cochlear nuclei are damaged."

Gerrard (1952), in a second paper, reported additional material, including the results of a questionnaire analysis of both Rh-incompatibility cases and prematurity cases. In this paper, he again emphasized the normal findings in the temporal bones of erythroblastotic neonates and the definitive finding of cochlear nuclear cellular destruction involving both dorsal and ventral cochlear nuclei. He also described frequent involvement of the floor of the fourth ventricle.

In 1956, as part of a Symposium on Rh deafness moderated by Dr. Hayes Newby, I summarized my data at that time as follows (Goodhill, 1956):

1. It is not the Rh factor alone which can produce kernicteric and cochlear nuclear lesions. The icteric lesion can be the sequel of isoimmunization by other serologic incompatibilities. Thus, there is evidence of ABO incompatibility and a new E serologic phenomenon as causes of erythroblastosis fetalis and its neurologic sequelae.

2. It is not the icterus alone which produces the lesions described. Rather, it is the cellular anoxia produced by icteric pigment deposition that actually destroys the integrity of the neural auditory pathway.

   Consequently, it now appears that cerebral hypoxia and anoxia, with or without icterus, can produce lesions in this area simulating lesions of kernicterus. It is not necessary for erythroblastosis fetalis to be present for cochlear nuclear lesions to occur.

3. Since the neurologic lesions are fairly haphazard and widespread, involvements of any portion of the neural auditory pathway may occur. Thus, the auditory sequelae may represent all sorts of combi-

nations of central lesions with the following variety of audiometric pictures.

a. There may be the simple central "nuclear deafness" described earlier which is a fairly fixed, stable, bilaterally symmetrical, neural hypacusis, usually moderate in degree, without recruitment, without tinnitus, and without peripheral vestibular involvement.

b. There may be a more complex type of greater degree with involvement of the central vestibular nuclei as well.

c. The neural auditory pathway may be involved in the thalamic and subcortical regions with the findings of neural dysacusis and many of the characteristics of aphasia. This group may include types which show both aphasic and nuclear components or aphasic components alone.

d. It is interesting to speculate on the possibility that the neurologic lesions may involve the reticular substance and the efferent cochlear pathway. Galambos (1954) and others consider that this efferent pathway may have a tuning effect on the cochlea. A disturbance of this type might explain the shifting thresholds and the wide disparity between pure-tone audiograms, speech thresholds, and speech discrimination scores in some of these patients.

e. The employment of the PGSR audiometric technique has shown interesting deviations in the cochlear nuclear case from the ordinary peripheral neural hypacusis case. The base line drifts and is fluctuant, the responses to shock are erratic, and the latent period is usually prolonged. The peaks are sharper and refractory and hyperactive phases occur. These differences in themselves are quite diagnostic in some cases and may point to a nuclear or more central lesion.

In the second decade following the discovery of the Rh factor, pediatric and hematologic advances in the treatment of erythroblastosis fetalis culminated in the development of exchange transfusions immediately after birth and after recognition of the lesion. In many cases, the needs for exchange transfusions were anticipated by careful quantitative studies of antibody titers in the Rh-negative mother. In addition to exchange transfusions, the obstetrical contributions to the treatment of the problem resulted in deliberately timed and carefully planned deliveries before term in an attempt to obviate the development of major erythroblastotic changes.

At a Symposium conducted by the American Academy of Cerebral Palsy in 1959, many of the leading authorities in the field of erythroblastosis fetalis gathered for a classic conference on this important subject. It is of great interest to note that Dr. William

Hardy, (1961) who took the responsibility for the audiologic evaluation of the problem at that conference, reported a very carefully studied group of Rh children in which he found "a divergent and complex state of affairs." This group of 48 children studied at the Johns Hopkins Audiologic Clinic revealed 17 aphasoid, 37 hypacusic children, and a number with mixed defects in hearing, language, and speech functions. The children ranged in age from 1.6 to 14 years.

Dr. Hardy stated that a number of these children behaved differently from children with ordinary peripheral auditory deficits, and he pointed out that not only were language disorders and dysarthria present in 22 percent of the children, but that a variety of sensory defects, some auditory and some quasi-auditory, were identified in this group of children. He stated that many of these children could tolerate loudness much better than ordinary peripheral sensorineural cases with similar audiograms.

At this same meeting, however, data were presented by two neuropathology groups, one from the Armed Forces Institute of Pathology headed by Dr. Webb Haymaker (1961), and another from the University of California, San Francisco, reported by Dr. Nathan Malamud (1961).

The Haymaker study from AFIP reported 80 cases of kernicterus and 7 cases of posticteric encephalopathy. *These studies were studies of brains only and did not include temporal bone examinations.* The brain studies, however, showed that the dorsal and ventral cochlear nuclei were always spared. Also unaffected were the trapezoid nucleus, the nucleus of the lateral lemniscus, and the medial geniculate body. The superior olivary nucleus sometimes contained a few necrotic nerve cells. The vestibular nuclei were damaged in many cases, but as a rule, relatively few nerve cells were necrotic.

Of the 7 cases of posticteric encephalopathy, 2 cases had definite histories of hearing loss. In the first case, that of a $6^{1}/_{2}$-month-old child with "apparent deafness," the medial geniculate body was normal. There was an atrophic pons and medulla, and there was an excess of glial fibers in the medial and lateral vestibular nuclei and also in the intramedullary fiber bundles of the vestibular nerve. The cochlear and trapezoid nuclei and the nuclei of the lateral lemniscus showed no changes, although the acoustic nerve seemed more gliosed than usual. Astrocytosis was very widespread in the pons and medulla, both in gray and white matter, involving cochlear nuclei, trapezoid body, lateral lemniscus, and reticular substance.

In the second case, that of a child of 3 years and 11 months with "defective hearing," the vestibular nuclei were affected, even though there was no history of clinical evidence of vestibular disturbance. Less affected were the trapezoid nuclei. There was some gliosis of the auditory nerve, and there was definite astrogliosis in the cochlear nuclei, trapezoid body, lateral lemniscus, and the white matter of the temporal lobe.

In commenting on the AFIP presentation, J. G. Greenfield of England speculated that the more mature a nerve cell, the more likely it is to undergo necrosis, since it has greater metabolic needs. He also pointed out that the brain stem was more severely damaged in kernicterus than in posticteric encephalopathy and that astrogliosis was an extremely important finding in these lesions. Greenfield indicated that there are a number of unexplained neuropathologic aspects in these cases as well as biochemical factors, e.g., in amino acids which may create toxic effects in auditory pathways not demonstrable by ordinary neuropathologic techniques. Again, it must be emphasized that no temporal bones were studied in this AFIP report. It should be noted, however, that in a number of the reports, damage to the reticular formation was mentioned, although without any particular significance attached to these descriptions.

Malamud's study also consisted of brains only, with no temporal-bone examinations. He found nothing in 10 brain autopsies of erythroblastotic children to explain deafness. Of his 10 cases, 7 died at the age of less than 1 year, and the others were ages 22, 32, and 55, all of whom were severely cerebral palsied and had very low I.Q.s. Consequently, although they did not have any communication, it is impossible to determine whether they really were "deaf."

We thus find an apparent beginning controversy in 1959 at the Academy of Cerebral Palsy meeting concerning the site of lesion.

Blakeley (1959), utilizing newer audiologic techniques, reported a series of 20 hearing-defective erythroblastotics (Rh athetoids) who were given tests of cochlear function in use at that time, namely, recruitment and aural-harmonic tests. The results demonstrated the presence of recruitment and a significantly reduced linear range of hearing in all the subjects. He concluded tentatively that the site of the injury in perceptive deafness associated with erythroblastosis is the cochlea. He also presented evidence at that time, on the basis of caloric tests, that vestibular function was essentially normal in $3/4$ of the ears tested. He also stated that the severity of hearing loss in erythroblastosis cannot be predicted from the severity of the associated athetosis.

Hyman and Keaster (1965) studied 372 hyperbilirubinemic neonates when the children reached the age of 4 years. As part of a comprehensive study of hyperbilirubinemic sequelae, oto-audiologic tests were performed. Thirteen (3.5 percent) of the 372 children had sensorineural hearing losses. In all, neonatal total serum bilirubin concentrations reached or exceeded 20 mg. percent. In two of the 13, maximum serum indirect bilirubin concentration was less than 20 mg. percent. Eleven of the 13 showed no neurologic abnormalities other than hearing loss, one had athetosis, and one a history of convulsions.

Studies by others, including Flottorp, Morley and Skatvedt (1957), Flower, Viehweg and Ruzicka (1966), and a recent doctoral dissertation by Matkin (1965), seem to point to end-organ involvement insofar as the site of lesion is concerned.

Matkin, in a summary of his dissertation, stated the following:

The predominate pattern of audiological findings from the special auditory tests was one most frequently encountered for individuals having cochlear damage. Specifically, SISI scores were positive and fixed-frequency Bekesy tracings were Type II at the higher frequencies. Further, the majority of the loudness balances indicated the presence of loudness recruitment, while tone decay was modest across frequency. In addition, most of the simultaneous binaural localizations were achieved when pure-tones of equivalent intensity were adjusted at the two ears.

Bizarre binaural summation which the writer had speculated might result from a central dysfunction was not reflected by the binaural threshold measurements. Another finding which did not appear to indicate central auditory damage was the fact that 77 percent of the subjects were successfully conditioned for electrodermal audiometry. Furthermore, the threshold responses recorded did not differ substantially from those obtained by routine pure-tone audiometry.

Although the audiological test results obtained in this study must be interpreted as indicating cochlear dysfunction, the inference of an end-organ lesion in this instance does not rule out the possibility that a more central aberration also exists in the hearing mechanism of the Rh subject. It must be remembered that prior research has indicated that central auditory deficits may not be apparent from auditory responses to pure-tone stimuli.

In a recent extensive audiologic investigation of four cases by Dr. Donald Dirks in our laboratory, findings similar to Matkin's were obtained. These findings will be reported in detail elsewhere.

As informal audiologic speculations begin to point to the cochlea as the primary site of lesion, hypoxia becomes a possible explanation for the bilateral audiologic symmetry which had previously been considered fairly good evidence for the existence of a central pathologic lesion.

Hypoxia and anoxia appear to be tenable hypotheses to explain symmetrical pure-tone cochlear lesions in these cases, particularly since recent auditory theory points to the unlikely production by brain-stem auditory lesions of pure-tone losses with maintenance of reasonably good speech discrimination.

At this point, however, this site-of-lesion mystery story becomes particularly interesting when one examines the experimental and clinical studies of Jens Hall (1964) in Norway, who conducted a major investigation (1) to examine histologically the pathological changes in fatal cases of asphyxia neonatorum, with particular reference to the organ of Corti and the cochlear nuclei; (2) to demonstrate the quality and the quantity of these changes; and (3) to evaluate whether the changes observed might reasonably explain the loss of hearing found in surviving cases.

Hall studied both brains and temporal bones of the human material as well as that of the experimental material. He concluded that the cochlear nuclei showed major qualitative and quantitative changes, the qualitative changes being characterized by degenerations ranging from nerve-cell contour blurring and peripheral nuclear displacements to vacuolization of the cytoplasm, loss of the nucleus, and total disintegration. As a result of these qualitative findings, he made a very meticulous quantitative examination of the cochlear nuclei and devised a method for counting the number of nerve cells in the cochlear nuclei. He found that there was a marked reduction in cochlear nuclei cell count in asphyxiated cases, the quantitative degree of cellular reduction approximating quite closely the duration of the asphyxia. He found that the dorsal cochlear nucleus was more heavily affected than the ventral, particularly in his human material. He attributes the cochlear nuclear damage to the fact that the cochlear nuclei represent the most richly vascularized areas of the brain stem.

As we ponder this fascinating game of oto-audiological, neuro-pathological, and otopathological dialectical ping-pong, we must not lose sight of the fact that to date not even one report has appeared of a case of hyperbilirubinemia with or without demonstrable kernicterus clinically in whom good audiologic studies are available and in which both temporal bone and neuropathologic studies have been carried out!

A recent communication from Dr. Raymond Carhart, whose chapter follows this one, makes some observations that are very startling in regard to auditory findings in brain-stem lesions. This is a most ingenious interpretation of psychoacoustic data and a major contribution to auditory theory insofar as the central auditory nervous system is concerned. I shall leave the details of this presentation to Dr. Carhart.

As we ponder the site-of-lesion dilemma, however, what in the meantime has happened to the Rh baby? Here we must bow in great humility to the obstetricians and pediatricians as we enter the era of fetal transfusions and spectrophotometric analysis of amniotic fluid. Today the Rh-negative mother who is suspected of having an Rh-positive fetus can be studied during the latter part of pregnancy by "trans-abdominal amniocenteses," carried out serially.

Starting at 20 weeks, amniotic fluid is obtained under local anesthesia through an abdominal needle puncture. This fluid is subjected to centrifugation and spectrophotometric scanning. An optical density wavelength chart is plotted. Criteria now are being standardized to guide the obstetrical plan of action, these spectrophotometric data being correlated with antibody titers. Delivery timing, indications for fetal transfusion, and exchange transfusions now are based to a large extent on biochemical information. In addition to these startling advances, it appears that development of an anti-Rh gamma globulin, which could be given prophylactically, is imminent.

Even without these newer advances, which obviously will diminish the incidence of post-hyperbilirubinemic hearing losses, we already are noting a marked decrease in auditory as well as neurologic sequelae of this disease. We have, indeed, come a long way from "septic jaundice of the newborn" to amniocentesis and fetal transfusions. We may thus look forward to almost complete abolition of Rh deafness as a clinical entity, so that perhaps in the future Rh deafness may well enter that group of iatrogenic auditory diseases previously described by Dr. Hawkins. These would be iatrogenic, not because of acts of commission, but because of acts of omission.

Epilogue

As we begin to study these cases with the greater sophistication now available with special auditory tests, including discrete frequency and sweep Bekesy tracings, SISI studies, loudness-balance tests, and tone-decay tests, we must not lose sight of the fact that the new cases we are seeing, fortunately less commonly, represent, in general, a much milder group of hyperbilirubinemias than those originally studied in the late 1940s and early 1950s. We are thus not really looking at the same disease; the etiology is similar, but the severity of complications has been greatly decreased.

Let us return, therefore, to the title of this chapter, "Auditory Pathway Lesions Resulting from Rh Factor Incompatibility." Where are we at this writing? As far as I can tell, we must continue to be very tentative in our assigning a site or sites of lesions. These cases demonstrate a wide spectrum of possible anatomic sites involving the cochlea (maybe?), the cochlear nuclei (?), probably the efferent (olivocochlear) pathway, possibly the reticular system, as well as geniculate, thalamic, and cortical areas. The fusion of knowledge of the newer audiology with the remarkable strides in the newer temporal-bone pathology, combined with the collaboration of our colleagues in neuropathology, will surely begin to take us somewhat closer to the answers.

References

Beneke, R. 1907. "Ueber den Kernikterus der Nuegeborenen." *München. med. Wchnschr.* **54**:2023–2027.

Bertrand, I. 1946. "Lesions du systeme nerveux central dans deux cas d'ictere nucleaire du nouveau-ne." *Rev. d'hemat.* **1**:399–420.

Blakeley, R. W. 1959. "Erythroblastosis and Perceptive Hearing Loss Responses of Athetoids to Tests of Cochlear Function." *J. Speech & Hearing Research,* **2**:5–15.

Coquet, M. 1944. "Les sequelles neurologiques tardives de l'ictere nucleaire." *Ann. paediat.* **163**:83–104.

Crabtree, N., and J. Gerrard. 1950. "Perceptive Deafness Associated with Severe Neonatal Jaundice." *J. Laryng. & Otol.* **64**:482–506.

Flottorp, G., D. E. Morley, and M. Skatvedt. 1957. "The Localization of Hearing Impairment in Athetoids." *Acta oto-laryng.* **48**:404–414.

Flower, R. M., R. Viehiveg, and W. R. Ruzicka. 1966. "The Communicative Disorders of Children with Kernicteric Athetosis: I. Auditory Disorders." *J. Speech & Hearing Disorders*, **31**:41–59.

Galambos, R. 1954. "Neural Mechanisms of Audition." *Physiol. Rev.* **34**:497–528.

Gerrard, J. 1952. "Nuclear Jaundice and Deafness." *J. Laryng. & Otol.* **66**:39–46.

Goodhill, V. 1947. "The Educational Treatment of the Pre-School Deaf Child. *Laryngoscope* **57**:555–563.

Goodhill, V. 1950. "Nuclear Deafness and the Nerve-Deaf Child: The Importance of the Rh Factor." *Tr. Am. Acad. Ophth. & Otolaryng.* **57**:671–687.

Goodhill, V. 1956. "Rh Child: Deaf or Aphasic? 1. Clinical and Pathological Aspects of Kernicteric Nuclear Deafness." *J. Speech & Hearing Disorders.* **21**:407–410.

Hall, J. 1964. "Cochlea and the Cochlear Nuclei in Asphyxia." *Acta oto-laryng. Suppl.* **194**.

Hardy, W. 1961. "Auditory Deficits of the Kernicterus Child." *American Academy for Cerebral Palsy, Kernicterus and Its Importance in Cerebral Palsy.* Springfield, Illinois: Charles C Thomas.

Haymaker, W. 1961. "Pathology of Kernicterus and Posticteric Encephalopathy." *American Academy for Cerebral Palsy, Kernicterus and Its Importance in Cerebral Palsy.* Springfield, Illinois: Charles C Thomas.

Hyman, C. B., and J. Keaster. 1965. "Personal Communication."

Landsteiner, K., and A. S. Wiener. 1940. "An Agglutinable Factor in Human Blood Serum Recognized by Immune Sera for Rhesus Blood." *Proc. Soc. Exper. Biol. & Med.* **43**:223.

Malamud, N. 1961. "Pathogenesis of Kernicterus in the Light of its Sequelae." *American Academy for Cerebral Palsy, Kernicterus and Its Importance in Cerebral Palsy.* Springfield, Illinois: Charles C Thomas.

Matkin, N. 1965. "Audiological Patterns Characterizing Hearing Impairments due to Rh Incompatibility." Doctoral dissertation. Northwestern University.

Orth, J. 1875. "Uber das Vorkommen von Bilirubinkrystallen bei neuge-
borenen Kinden." *Arch. path. Anat.* **63**:447–462.

Phelps, W. 1941. "The Management of the Cerebral Palsies. *J.A.M.A.*
117:1621–1625.

Potter, Edith. 1947. "Rh—Its Relation to Congenital Hemolytic Disease
and to Intra-Group Transfusion Reactions." Chicago, Illinois: Year
Book Publishing Co.

Schmorl, C. G. 1904. "Zur Kenntniss des Ikterus neonatorum, insbe-
sondere der dabei auftretenden Gehirnveranderungen, *Verhandl,
deutsch, path. Gesellsch.* **15**:109–115.

AUDIOLOGIC TESTS:
QUESTIONS AND SPECULATIONS

IN this chapter, I shall examine the hypothesis that there probably are lesions of the central auditory system which, when tested audiologically, mimic cochlear lesions in many respects and which, in consequence, are commonly misjudged to be peripheral hearing impairments. One implication of this hypothesis is that such audiological findings as positive SISI scores, Type II Bekesy tracings, and recruitment can appear when the inner ear is normal but when lower sections of the central auditory system (particularly the cochlear nuclei) are damaged.

Let no one misunderstand. Inner ear lesions ordinarily lead to the constellation of test results just mentioned. The point at issue is whether this same constellation can also appear when an appropriate retrocochlear lesion has occurred. The hypothesis under scrutiny states that it can.

This chapter briefly reviews the issues in question as these issues are exemplified by persons with hearing losses due to erythroblastosis fetalis and kernicterus.

Persons with hearing losses classifiable under this cause almost always exhibit some degree of athetosis or rigidity (Perlstein, 1961). Moreover, many of the individuals with history of brain injury associated with neonatal jaundice exhibit auditory imperceptions which Perlstein (1961) describes as "impressive auditory aphasia," and Hardy (1961) speaks of it as "perceptive-associative difficulties." Both these men have however pointed out, as have

229

others (Crabtree and Gerrard, 1950; Flower, *et al.*, 1966; Gerrard, 1952; Goodhill, 1950; and Rosen, 1956) that hearing loss in the traditional sense is a frequent sequel to neonatal jaundice.

Several investigators have explored systematically the hearing losses arising from kernicterus. The results, if one limits oneself to consideration of data from patients mature enough to be capable of giving consistent responses, are in reasonable agreement. Their pure-tone audiograms typically exhibit relatively close bilateral symmetry, only a mild loss for low frequencies, but substantial loss at high frequencies. Within this frame of reference, individual configurations vary in degree and detail. As can be seen from Table I, however, the group audiograms obtained in

TABLE I

CENTRAL TENDENCIES OF PURE-TONE THRESHOLDS (RE ISO 1964 NORMS) EXHIBITED BY SAMPLE OF PATIENTS WITH HEARING LOSSES DUE TO KERNICTERUS. RESULTS FOR THE TWO EARS COMBINED WHERE POSSIBLE. VALUES FOR BLAKELEY AND MATKIN 1 EXTRACTED FROM PUBLISHED AUDIOGRAMS. MEDIANS FOR FLOWER **ET AL.** COMPUTED BY PRESENT WRITER. MATKIN 1 DATA GLEANED BY HIM FROM CLINIC FILES AT NORTH-WESTERN. MATKIN 1 DATA OBTAINED BY HIM ON A SECOND POPULATION.

Study	N	Test Frequency						
		125	250	500	1000	2000	4000	8000
Blakely[a]	20		30	42	55	68.5	74	81.5
Flower, **et al.**[c]	15		32.5	40.5	60.8	65.0	79.7	
Hardy[b]	26		33.2	38.4	45.7	53.8	56.4	
Matkin 1[a]	40	29	33	45	63	70.5	74	74.5
Matkin 2[c]	22	29.3	31.8	49.3	68.4	76.0	77.5	73.5

a. Approximate mean estimated from Matkin's (1965) figures.
b. Mean.   c. Median.

the major studies are very similar, and they bespeak a characteristic clinical entity (Blakeley, 1959; Flower, *et al.*, 1966; Hardy, 1961; and Matkin, 1965). The characteristic configuration is one with ISO 1964 thresholds as follows: about 30 dB for 125 and 250 cps, about 40 dB for 500 cps, about 60 dB for 1,000 cps, and about 70 dB for 2,000 cps, about 75 dB for 4,000 cps and about 75 dB for 8,000 cps. Acuity for speech has not been studied as extensively, but speech reception thresholds have been found to agree rather well with the average pure-tone acuity in the mid-frequencies (Flower, et al., 1966, and Matkin, 1965). Speech discrimination is variable (Matkin, 1965), but the noteworthy feature is that it often may be very good (Flottorp, et al., 1957, and Hardy, 1961).

Blakeley (1959) as well as Flottorp, et al. (1957) found kernic-teric patients to experience recruitment. Blakeley also found that they underwent aural overload at low sensation levels. Blake-ley's findings led him to conclude tentatively that "the site of injury in perceptive deafness associated with erythroblastosis fetalis is in the cochlea." Matkin (1965) confirmed the presence of recruitment. He also found that at high frequencies SISI scores were positive and Bekesy tracings were Type II. He states that "in terms of audiological thinking one must reach the con-clusion that Rh incompatibility induces inner-ear damage when it results in a hearing loss."

Matkin adds the thought that there may be "a dual dysfunction of the auditory system resulting from hyperbilirubinemia. This involves damage at both the levels of the cochlea and the cen-tral auditory pathways." He thus takes cognizance of the fact that kernicterus often produces harm to the auditory system within and above the brain stem, but he implies that such lesions do not bring about the recruitment, positive SISI scores and Type II Bekesy tracings he observed.

One can not question the test findings, but the interpretation that they indicate cochlear lesions is contradictory to a widely held opinion that the auditory deficits of kernicteric-athetotics are not a result of inner-ear impairment. According to this opinion, the peripheral sensorineural mechanism is presumed to have escaped damage, while auditory centers within the central nervous system are presumed to have been harmed (Byers, et al., 1955; Goodhill, 1956; Hardy, 1961; Newby, 1964; and Perlstein, 1961). Hardy (1961), for example, said, "There is no evidence, as yet, that there is any causal relationship between kernicterus asso-ciated with the Rh factor and lesions of the conductive and receptive stages of the auditory system. Lesions may exist here concurrently, but it is . . . at the level of the auditory nuclei, low in the pons . . . that the lesion relating to kernicterus has been identified." He added that higher segments of the auditory path-ways may be involved. Clearly, if kernicterus tends to spare the cochlear system (except as such lesion may result from unrelated happenstance, as Hardy's statement implies), one must seek a non-peripheral mechanism responsible for recruitment, positive SISI scores and Type II tracings.

In contemplating these issues, one must take cognizance of the evidence Dr. Goodhill has presented. Remember that a number of postmortem studies have shown that kernicteric foci in the cochlear nuclei are common as part of the kernicteric involvement of the central nervous system (Bertrand, 1946; Crabtree and Gerrard, 1950; Dublin, 1951; and Gerrard, 1952), although some contradictory evidence also has been presented (Haymaker, et al., 1961, and Malamud, 1961). It has been observed that other portions of the central auditory tract also are frequently affected. By contrast, except for the somewhat doubtful case reported by Kelemen (1956), postmorten exploration has not similarly demonstrated cochlear damage (Crabtree and Gerrard, 1950; Gerrard, 1952; and Goodhill, 1956).

The reasonable conclusion in the light of the foregoing evidence is that any child with hearing disorders caused by kernicterus probably possesses lesions within the cochlear nuclei and also possibly elsewhere in the central auditory system. In such event, the auditory peculiarities exhibited by this child must be due either 1) to concomitant inner-ear damage which is masking the symptomatology of the deeper lesion 2) or else the auditory signs arise in consequence of the central lesions per se. There is no reason to expect the aforementioned peripheral masking of central symptomatology. Moreover, since the likelihood of inner-ear damage is less than that of central damage, the latter must often occur alone. In such event, whatever symptomatology is distinctive with central damage should then appear, even if masking by a cochlear lesion were to occur when such a lesion was also present. Thus, the more parsimonious alternative is to reason that audiological findings such as reported by Blakeley (1959) and Matkin (1965) are in consequence of CNS damage.

This latter view is the hypothesis posed at the outset of the present paper: that the typical syndrome of high-tone audiometric loss, recruitment, positive SISI scores, and type II Bekesy tracings evidenced by kernicteric-athetotics with hearing loss results when normal trains of information from the inner ear suffer disruption in transmission through damaged cochlear nuclei and/or associated basal centers en route to perceptual processing in higher centers.[1]

The evidence supporting this hypothesis is still tenuous at some points, but it is nonetheless sufficient to warrant consideration. The question at hand involves finding a reconciliation that can explain the generation of the audiological syndrome in consequence of abnormalities of central functioning. The remainder of this paper is concerned with this question.

The audiogram which typifies kernicteric hearing loss has already been described (see Table I). It exhibits a pattern which when examined carefully is distinctive. This configuration is illustrated in Figure I, which plots the median audiogram for Matkin's (1965) research subjects. Note that this audiogram possesses three regions. Acuity is relatively good from 250 cps down. It is uniformly poor for high frequencies. Between these two regions there is a fairly uniform transition, but the greatest change appears across the octave from 500 to 1000 cps.

One must conclude from this audiogram that the kernicteric lesion producing it is frequency selective in a unique way. We have here a high tone loss similar but not identical to the patterns exhibited rather commonly by other types of patients with sensorineural involvements. The matter that must be now clarified is whether losses of this general pattern may at times arise from damage in the cochlear nuclei, and/or adjacent auditory centers where postkernicteric lesions are likely, instead of always arising from more peripheral pathology.

At this point we must remind ourselves of Wever's (1949) Volley-Place theory, which stresses that the normal auditory system has two mechanisms for response in the frequency domain. The volley mechanism embodies sensitivity to the number of bursts of neural excitation occurring per unit time, while the place mechanism yields sensitivity to the locus on the basilar membrane undergoing maximum excursion. According to Wever's theory, the two mechanisms function concomitantly over a wide range of intermediate frequencies with only volley operating in response to very low frequencies and only place

---

1. This hypothesis does not contradict the expectation that other symptoms, characteristic of auditory imperception, will appear when major lesions occur at still higher levels, either alone or in combination with lower-level lesions of the type under discussion here.

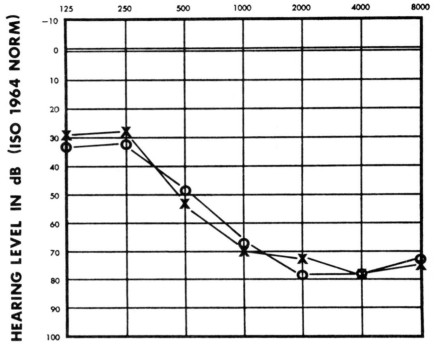

Figure 1. Median audiograms for the right and left ears of 22 subjects with hearing impairments resulting from Rh incompatibility. (Plotted re ISO 1964 norm) (Matkin, 1965)

operating for very high ones. The theory implies that there is a decrease in the importance of each mechanism in the transition away from the range where it is of primary significance.

The Volley-Place theory has not been popular in recent years, and clinicians have not often asked themselves what its practical implications might be. Instead, they have based their thinking on the modern version of the Place Theory. The potential role of the volley mechanism has been minimized as workers have contemplated Bekesy's (1960) analyses of the mechanical action of the cochlear partition; Bekesy's emphasis on differential inhibition, sharpening and funneling of afferent information by the nervous system; and the extensive evidence from electrophysiology that individual neurons in the eighth nerve and the cochlear nuclei have characteristic frequencies to which they are most sensitive (Katsuki, et al., 1962; Kiang, et al., 1962, 1965; Rose,

1960; and Tasaki, 1960). Only fleeting emphasis has been given to such observations as that only a very few single units with characteristic frequencies below 300 cps have been found within the eighth nerve, that the lowest of these characteristic frequencies are in the 110–125 cps range, and that neural discharge maintains good synchrony with individual sound waves throughout a broad range of lower frequencies (Katsuki, et al., 1962; Kiang, et al., 1962; Tasaki, 1960; and Wever, 1949). As Kiang, et al. (1962) put it on the basis of single-unit responses to clicks, "the unit fires only at discrete times that correspond to a particular phase of displacement of the basilar membrane." They emphasize that true volleying (i.e., many discharges in synchrony with one another) arises only from units linked to the basal turn of the cochlea, but one must nonetheless conclude that units linked to middle and apical portions of the cochlea exhibit synchrony individually even though they are not in step as a group.[2] The end result, considering the entire network of cochlea innervation, is that timing information is preserved in the discharge pattern of many neurons, even though their composite firing is not the most obvious form of volleying. This timing information is in addition to any place information which arises because of the site of major agitation on the basilar membrane.

Emerging evidence may modify details of the Volley-Place theory but the critical consideration for our discussion is the fact that the theory allows for two processes underlying tonal perception. This latitude is particularly important when one recalls that a "periodicity pitch" mechanism can be demonstrated through psychological experiments. For example, there is Schouten's (1962) and Ritsma's work (1962) on the pitch residue, the investigations by Small and his associates (Small and Campbell, 1961; Thurlow and Small, 1955) with pulsed tones, and various studies with repeated bursts of noise (Harris, 1963; Miller and Taylor, 1948; and Nieder and Creelman, 1965). Licklider (1959, 1962) has been particularly active in developing models to account for recoding by the central auditory mechanism of the information carried by the time pattern of the output from the cochlea. Bekesy (1963) stated that the periodicity theory as formulated by Schouten and Licklider "has no difficulties in the

2. It is not implied that each unit will fire with every incoming wave, but only that when firing does occur it is initiated in that unit at approximately the same phase of the wave.

lower frequency range, but it encounters some problems in higher frequencies." Finally, Davis *et al.* (1951), in discussing their own experiment with low-frequency pulsing of a high frequency tone, stated, "*frequencies* above 4,000 cps (and probably all available frequencies) are translated in the ear into *position,* i.e., to *choice of channel;* but below 800 cps (and perhaps, but the volley principle, up to 4,000 cps) information as to frequency is *also* carried in the form of *time-interval between impulses....* It now seems clear that either place or frequency or both may be the physiological correlate(s) of physical frequency."

Licklider (1959, 1962) makes eminently clear that the decoding of periodicity information must occur central to the eighth nerve. Likewise, the sharpening and funneling of place information described by Bekesy (1960) must occur within the central nervous system. Thus, two independent analyzing processes, one for volley and one for place, must normally proceed concurrently. Moreover, these analyses must undergo at least their first stage of differentiation within the cochlear nuclei. These nuclei are clearly complicated sorting stations rather than merely relay points for neural excitation. In all probability the neural networks within the cochlear nuclei that are responsible for the volley-analyzing process are dissimilar to the networks serving the place-identifying process, i.e., the two may well involve relatively independent arrays of neural tissue within the cochlear nuclei. Thus, at the level of these nuclei the stage is set for differential disruption of the volley-sensing mechanism as contrasted to interference with the place-sensing mechanism. The same may be said for subsequent centers within the central auditory tract, provided the two processes continue to be neurologically distinctive.

Bearing these considerations in mind, one may postulate that kernicteric damage in the cochlear nuclei (and/or possibly other lower centers of the auditory system) disrupts the volley-sensitive mechanism much less than the place-sensitive one. The end result would be an audiometric configuration of the general form shown in Figure 1.

The concepts involved are illustrated in Figure 2. Parameters for this illustration are arbitrary, but they were chosen to yield a configuration conforming closely to the median-audiogram Matkin obtained. Here the volley mechanism is considered as being impaired about 30 dB (ISO 1964) and the place mechanism about 75 dB. The transitional range within which the volley mech-

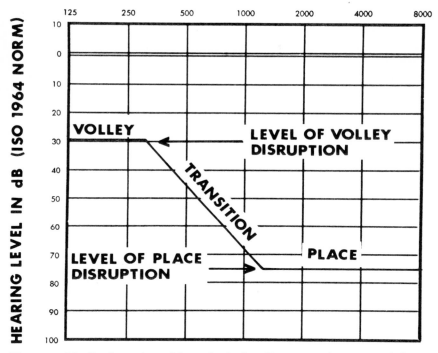

Figure 2. Idealized version of hypothetical audiogram to be expected from 30 dB interference with volley-sensing mechanism and 75 dB interference with place-sensing mechanism.

anism becomes progressively less efficient is envisioned here as beginning at 300 cps and terminating at 1300 cps, where the place mechanism is presumed to predominate sufficiently to be the sole determinant of threshold.

The foregoing line of thought may be restated as follows: a lesion producing differential disruption in acuity as postulated in Figure 2 must be situated at or beyond the site where neurological decoding separates volley information from place information. It must also be situated at a site where postkernicteric damage will disrupt one information-sensing mechanism more than the other. There is little prospect that this site is within the inner ear or the eighth nerve. These structures are not likely to be differentially harmed by kernicterus; but even if they were, place information and volley information are simultaneously captured here in one complex pattern of neural discharge whose details depend simultaneously upon the number of neurons active and the relative synchrony of excitation of each. Full separation of the two sets of information must be delayed until neural centers are reached where differentiated decoding and distinctive recoding can take place.

The cochlear nuclei are the first centers where this separation may be presumed to occur. Without attempting to assign particular functions to particular portions of this neural complex, recall that a neat tonotopic (place) distribution has been demonstrated within the cochlear nuclei but that this distribution covers only higher frequencies. Very low frequencies, if one may judge from experimentation on the cat (Rose, 1960), are not tied to tonotopic mapping, and such mapping appears sparse for frequencies below 700–800 cps.

The foregoing considerations give credence to the hypothesis that the person with hearing loss resulting from kernicterus ordinarily has *normal inner-ear and eighth-nerve function* but that damage within his cochlear nuclei disturbs transmission of information beyond these nuclei. Moreover, according to this hypothesis the mechanism for place-sensing is considered the more impaired.[3]

The foregoing discussion suggests the manner in which the audiogram of kernicterus may be attributed to non-peripheral lesions, but a second hypothesis is needed to account for the triad of recruitment, positive SISI scores (at high frequencies) and Type II Bekesy tracings which kernicterics demonstrate. This second hypothesis is simple. It postulates that even though the person with kernicteric hearing loss is not aware of low-level sounds, his experiences soon after the sound exceeds his threshold will approximate normal auditory experience for stimulation at the same intensity level. Here the assumption is that the kernicteric

3. An alternate possibility must be recognized. It is not clear whether the volley mechanism, though it can be demonstrated to operate, normally takes precedence over place at any frequency. That is, even for low frequencies the volley mechanism may have a poorer threshold than does the place mechanism. In such event, the configuration in Figure 2 could result from disturbance of only the place-sensing mechanism. The minor deficit depicted in the figure at low frequencies would then represent the unimpaired sensitivity of the volley-sensing system. This alternative does not change the hypothesis that the functioning of the inner ear and eighth nerve are normal following kernicteric damage to hearing while the functioning of the cochlear nuclei is not.

lesion acts primarily to block transmission of low-intensity information through the cochlear nuclei but that a gating effect operates so that signals that exceed thresholds appreciably have about the same ultimate effect subjectively as in the absence of kernicteric damage. Remember that the processes that will go on within the cochlear nuclei, even when these are impaired, will be highly complex. Moreover, neural signals reaching these nuclei will not vary linearly with changing intensity, either in the number of activated neurons or in the rate of their firings. In view of these facts, it is highly improbable that a fixed decibel deficit will be maintained by the kernicteric patient at all stimulus intensities. The more likely outcome would seem to be that the cochlear nuclei exhibit a gating action which, soon after threshold is exceeded, allows auditory experience to become nearly normal for the intensity level being employed.

According to this view, the behavior to be expected when an auditory test is administered to a person with kernicteric hearing loss is determined primarily by the intensity level at which the test is administered rather than by the sensation level of the presentation. Sensation level enters the picture only to the extent that testing conditions are specified in terms of it.

On this basis, the question of whether a patient's response is peripherally aberrant must be answered in terms of whether a normal hearer presented with the same task at the same intensity level would have behaved in the same manner.

When we apply this point of view to the syndrome of special test results exhibited by persons with kernicteric hearing loss, their responses may be considered as approximately normal for the intensity level at which these tests must be given to them. In other words, the recruitment, positive SISI scores, and Type II Bekesy tracings that characterize this syndrome are consistent with the hypothesis that individuals with kernicteric hearing loss possess fully normal peripheral systems (end-organ and eighth nerve) coupled with nuclear lesions that block awareness of faint-level stimuli but that allow unimpaired response to higher levels. Remember, that when these tests are administered, the patient's threshold deficit at each frequency will determine the intensity at which special audiological tests are presented to him, and his behavior can be expected to change from one frequency to another when the presentation level is shifted substantially in consequence of his audiometric contour.

To clarify this line of reasoning, let us analyze first the fact that persons with kernicteric hearing loss exhibit recruitment when tested by the Reger monaural balance method. Figure 3 illustrates how this could come about without cochlear involvement. The figure carries at its base of reference the median thresholds of Matkin's subjects. The monaural balance test was administered by setting the more impaired frequency of the two being compared at a sensation level of 20 dB and adjusting the second frequency to the same loudness. Both stimuli were at high presentation levels. Now, assuming that there is a gating process operating within the cochlear nuclei, the result would be that both tones would evoke a very substantial loudness simply because such loudness is normal at these intensity levels. The crucial point, however, is that according to the hypothesis that suprathreshold responses are nearly normal, in the process of balancing the two signals to the same loudness, the second tone would have been varied until the two signals lay on the same normal contour of equal loudness. Each half of Figure 3 shows two points on this loudness contour. These points are labeled Theoretical Normal, and they represent the balance that would have occurred had the two stimuli been balanced by a normal hearing subject. Chart A depicts this normal balance for a 250–500 cps match. It also shows the median balance obtained for this match by Matkin's subjects. Chart B shows the same items for the 250–1000 cps match. It is immediately apparent from the figure that Matkin's findings must be described as showing "recruitment" in that the slope between frequencies found in the threshold curve was not retained during the bi-frequency loudness balance; but there is no evidence here that the observed results appeared because of end-organ damage. Unimpaired end-organ function and central gating could also yield as much "recruitment."

Figure 4 illustrates that positive scores might at times merge from a standard SISI test without there being an inner-ear lesion. Here Chart A, on the left, merely depicts the series of test conditions being considered in this illustration. This chart, too, carries the median threshold audiogram for Matkin's group. SISI tests, when administered in the presence of these amounts of

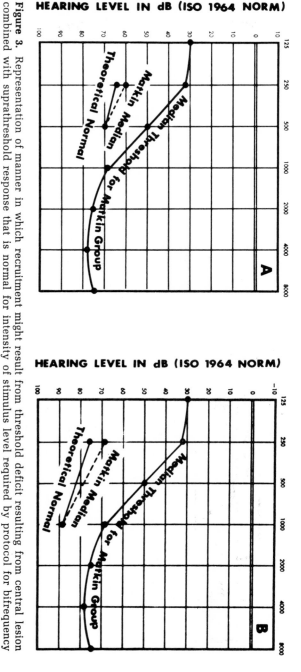

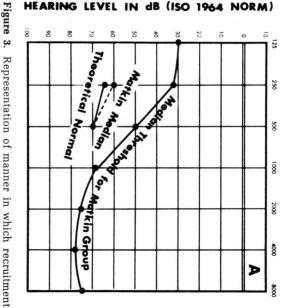

Figure 3. Representation of manner in which recruitment might result from threshold deficit resulting from central lesion combined with suprathreshold response that is normal for intensity of stimulus level required by protocol for bifrequency monoaural loudness balance test (see text for detail).

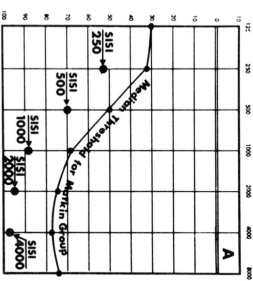

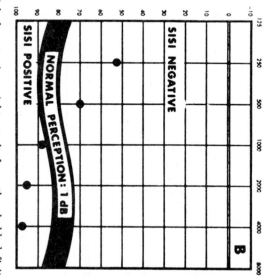

Figure 4. Representation of manner in which positive SISI scores at high frequencies might result from threshold deficit resulting from central lesion combined with suprathreshold response that is normal for intensity of stimulus level required by protocol for SISI test (see text for detail).

hearing loss, required presentation levels 20 dB stronger, as depicted by the series of arrows and filled circles in Chart A. The filled circles are reproduced anew in Chart B, at the right. Note that some of them fall above and others fall below the band labeled "NORMAL PERCEPTION: 1 dB." This band, which undulates across the chart, is the estimated boundary between the hearing level at which normal auditors may be expected to achieve positive SISI scores with regularity and fainter levels, where the anticipated percentages would usually be too poor to be classed as positive. This boundary is positioned as shown here in consequence of Thompson's (1963) report of Young's work on detection of 1 dB increments by normal listeners, but Young's observation has been transferred to the ISO scale and is depicted as a band 10 dB wide.

Recognizing that this basis for specifying the boundary for normal perception of 1 dB increments is approximate at best, the figure nonetheless epitomizes graphically the fact that SISI tests given to normal listeners at levels reaching and exceeding this boundary will result in a very high percentage of increment identification, while tests given at substantially fainter levels will not. It follows, if this premise is correct, that SISI tests given to normal hearers at the levels shown in Chart B by the filled circles would not be consistently positive at 250 or 500 cps, because these levels are not intense enough to reach "NORMAL PERCEPTION: 1 dB." By contrast, the test levels for 1,000, 2,000 and 4,000 cps are high enough to fall in the region where normals should ordinarily obtain positive SISI scores.

Since it was only at these latter frequencies that Matkin found the SISI scores of kernicteric subjects to be positive, one is again faced with a situation wherein the test results yielded by Matkin's group parallel results normal listeners would give when tested at the same intensity levels. Such an outcome clearly does not allow one to conclude that Matkin's subjects exhibited abnormality of response on the SISI test or that they gave positive SISI scores because they possessed inner-ear lesions. One can just as logically reason that through action of a gating function the stimulus level was sufficiently high to evoke a fully normal set of responses despite a limitation in the ability of these persons to perceive lower stimuli satisfactorily. Stated another way, positive SISI scores at the test levels required by the typical kernicteric subject are not unequivocal evidence of any peripheral abnormality in response.[4]

We come now to the question of Bekesy audiometry. The important consideration here is that during presentation of the continuous tone used in this type of test the intensity of the sustained stimulus within the inner ear will be great enough to cause peripheral adaptation provided the inner ear and eighth nerve are normal. That is, the equilibration phenomenon that Derbyshire (1934) described will come into play, the end result of which will be a drop in the activity within the auditory nerve. Such peripheral adaptation cannot help having a marked effect under circumstances where a fixed level of neural activity is necessary for response to penetrate beyond a central lesion that is causing a shift in the threshold of awareness. A listener with such a lesion will be able to maintain his perception of the tone only if the external stimulus is increased in intensity enough to compensate for the reduced neural activity which adaptation brings about.

Figure 5 shows how peripheral adaptation would lead to a Type II Bekesy tracing. Here we see two curves in Chart A. The upper one is the Matkin audiogram. The lower one is plotted below this audiogram by the amount of adaptation that, according to Jerger's (1957) work, one would predict that a normal listener would undergo after one minute of sustained exposure at the intensity levels depicted by the Matkin curve. The one-minute time boundary was chosen for use here because adaptation takes place preponderantly during the first minute. This lower curve thus traces the stimulus levels that would be needed for awareness to continue after one minute of stimulation when the peripheral sys-

4. In this regard, it is worth commenting that most of Matkin's subjects actually obtained SISI scores substantially lower than 100 percent in the circumstances where very high scores would be the expectation for normal hearers. At 1,000 cps, for example, only 5 of 22 scores exceeded 60 percent and two of these five were below 90 percent. Or, again, Matkin classified 18 scores at 4,000 cps as positive because he included any score of 65 percent or more in this category. Only seven of the 18 scores, however, were 90 percent or better, while another seven did not exceed 75 percent. Thus, viewed in the aggregate, Matkin's group was less sensitive to the 1 dB increments of the SISI test than normals would be at the same intensity level. It is hard to see how such results can be taken as unequivocal evidence of inner-ear lesions.

HEARING LEVEL IN dB (ISO 1964 NORM)

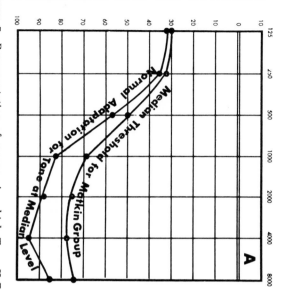

HEARING LEVEL IN dB (ISO 1964 NORM)

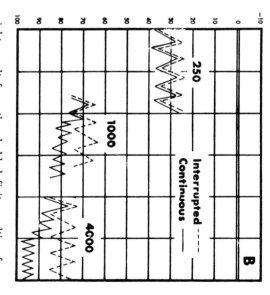

Figure 5. Representation of manner in which Type II Bekesy tracings might result from threshold deficit resulting from central lesion combined with peripheral adaptation during continuous tracing that is normal for intensity level at which threshold is traced (see text for detail).

tem is not impaired and when the threshold level is determined by central damage.

Chart B illustrates how this factor would affect fixed-frequency Bekesy tracings. It plots the curves for 250, 1,000 and 4,000 cps that one would predict if peripheral adaptation in the magnitudes pictured in Chart A were modifying the stimulus level required to maintain perception of the continuous tone. Note that the interrupted stimulus would not be subject to the adaptation effect because of the silent intervals it incorporates. Hence, its tracing is here shown as being maintained at the initial threshold level. The companion tracing for the continuous tone was started at the same level, but it was drawn to reach the adapted level at the end of a minute.[5] This second tracing was also drawn as narrowing whenever appreciable adaptation is depicted. The rationale for such narrowing is Endicott's (1964) observation that differential sensitivity is better in the adapted than the unadapted normal ear.[6]

The relationship to be seen in the three tracings in Chart B are clean-cut. The pattern for 250 cps is obviously Type I, whereas those for 1,000 and 4,000 cps are definitely Type II. Thus, in theory at least, Type II Bekesy tracings should result when normal peripheral adaptations coupled with centrally imposed loss in acuity at the presentation levels which kernicterics require when doing Bekesy tracings at 1,000 and 4,000 cps. Consequently, we find ourselves in the situation where the occurrence of a Type II Bekesy tracing can not always be accepted as evidence of inner-ear damage, any more than recruitment or positive SISI scores can be. We are faced for the third time with the situation wherein an audiological finding that is a typical

5. One need not be concerned by the fact that the continuous tone does not maintain a constant intensity when obtaining a Bekesy tracing with it, since when one assumes normal peripheral function, as we are doing here, the stimulus level will remain relatively high even during the time when it is not audible. Thus, despite its minor fluctuations, the stimulus will be ample as exposure continues to retain and to increase the peripheral adaptation. That is, it is irrelevant insofar as peripheral adaptation is concerned that the listener does not have continuous awareness of the test tone. What is pertinent is that his peripheral mechanism is not given any respite from stimulation.

6. It may be that Endicott's finding is not apropos to the present instance because it was observed at suprathreshold levels, but there is sufficient prospect of its applicability so that the adapted portion of each for the continuous tones was drawn with narrowed amplitude.

feature of kernicteric hearing impairment can as logically have its basis in a nuclear lesion than in a cochlear one.

The foregoing discussion is an abbreviated resume of some of the lines of thinking and some of the considerations which support the belief that kernicterus can produce a type of central auditory damage characterized by a definite hearing loss as measured audiometrically and by the configuration of other audiological findings conventionally interpreted as indicating inner-ear lesion. There are obviously many details that still remain to be learned about the effects kernicterus has on the newborn child, their influences on early behavior, and the principles for interpreting audiological tests. At the moment, the hypotheses outlined in this paper are as warranted as are their counter-hypotheses, which many audiologists favor. Neither view can currently be accepted with surety. Much research remains to be done. This research, rather than speculation, must be the first order of business. Meanwhile, however, the above views are presented here for two reasons. First, these views remind us that there is always danger of oversimplifying and habituating our interpretation of clinical tests. Secondly, they illustrate the opinion that there exist central auditory damages which mimic cochlear lesions audiologically, so that these particular conditions have been misjudged as peripheral hearing impairments. The evidence at my disposal leads me currently to the belief that postnatal kernicterus often fits this category.

In summary and conclusion, the foregoing discussion examines the hypothesis that kernicterus produces central auditory damages which when tested audiologically mimic cochlear lesions in many respects and which, in consequence, are often misdiagnosed as peripheral sensory impairments. One reason for concern with this hypothesis is that central damages from other causes may be susceptible to similar misdiagnosis, but this paper deals directly only with the question of kernicteric hearing loss.

We are faced with a paradox wherein postmortem evidence suggests that kernicterus produces lesions within the central nervous system, including the cochlear nuclei, while persons with kernicteric hearing loss show auditory behavior conventionally attributed to inner-ear lesion. The paradox can be resolved and the audiogram characterizing kernicteric hearing loss can be accounted for by making five assumptions: that the lesions involved are in the cochlear nuclei; that place information and volley information receive their first definitely separate coding within the cochlear nuclei; that lesions produced in these nuclei by kernicterus impede the mechanism for sensing and transmitting place information more than the mechanism serving volley information is impeded, thus giving rise to the audiometric configuration typical of post-kernicteric hearing loss; that stimulation vigorous enough to exceed appreciably these threshold levels activate a gating phenomenon which leads to auditory experiences that are approximately normal for the intensity level of the moment; that the inner ear is free from lesion so that its behavior will be normal for the intensity level being employed.

These assumptions allow the suprathreshold audiological behavior of kernicterics to be explained in the following manner. The recruitment demonstrable through monaural bifrequency loudness balance appears because the tones being compared align themselves on the same normal contour for equal loudness. SISI scores become positive at high frequencies simply because presentation levels at these frequencies are so intense that it is normal to perceive 1 dB increments consistently. Type II Bekesy tracings can be attributed to the changes in stimulus level required in consequence of the auditory adaptation that sustained stimulation evokes in a normal peripheral system.

Consequently, since it is not necessary to assume an inner-ear lesion as the reason for appearance of recruitment, positive SISI scores and Type II Bekesy tracings, and since other evidence favors the theory that kernicterus produces central lesions within the auditory system, it seems justifiable to reason, pending further research, that we have here an instance of central auditory disorder.

References

Bekesy, George von. 1960. Experiments in Hearing (trans. and ed. by G. Wever). New York: McGraw-Hill.

Bekesy, George von. 1963. "Hearing Theories and Complex Sounds." *J. Acoustical Soc. Am.*, **35**:588–601.

Bertrand, I. 1946. "Lesions due Systeme Nerveux Central Dans Deux Cas D'ictere du Nouveau-ne." *Rev. hemat.*, **1**:339–420.

Blakely, R. W. 1959. "Erythroblastosis and Hearing Loss: Responses of Athetoids to Tests of Cochlear Function." *J. Speech & Hearing Res.*, **2**:5–15.

Byers, R. K., R. S. Payne and B. Crothers. 1955. "Extrapyramidal Cerebral Palsy with Hearing Loss following Erythroblastosis." *Pediatrics*, **15**:248–254.

Crabtree, N., and J. Gerrard. 1950. "Perceptive Deafness Associated with Severe Neonatal Jaundice; Report of 16 Cases." *J. Laryngol. & Otol.*, **64**:482–506.

Davis, Hallowell, S. Richard Silverman and D. R. McAuliffe. 1951. "Some Observations on Pitch and Frequency," *J. Acoustical Soc. Am.*, **23**:40–42.

Derbyshire, Arthur J. 1934. "Action Potentials of the Auditory Nerve." Dissertation. Harvard University.

Dublin, W. 1951. "Neurological Lesions of Erythroblastosis Fetalis in Relation to Nuclear Deafness." *Am. J. Clin. Path.*, **21**:935–938.

Endicott, J. 1964. "The Influence of Auditory Adaptation on Differential Sensitivity to Intensity Change in Normal Ears." Ph.D. dissertation. Northwestern University.

Flottorp, G., D. E. Morley and M. Skatvedt. 1957. "The Localization of Hearing Impairment in Athetoids." *Acta oto-laryng.*, **48**:404–414.

Flower, R. M., R. Viehweg and W. R. Rizicka. 1966. "The Communicative Disorders of Children with Kernicteric Athetosis: I, Auditory Disorders." *J. Speech & Hearing Disorders*, **31**:41–59.

Gerrard, J. 1952. "Nuclear Jaundice and Deafness." *J. Laryng. & Otol.*, **66**:39–46.

Goodhill, Victor. 1950. "Nuclear Deafness and the Nerve-Deaf Child: the Importance of the Rh Factor." *Tr. Am. Acad. Ophth.*, **54**:671–687.

Goodhill, Victor. 1956. "Clinical Pathological Aspects of Kernicteric Nuclear 'Deafness'." *J. Speech & Hearing Disorders*, **21**:407–410.

Goodhill, Victor. 1957. "Pathology, Diagnosis and Therapy of Deafness." *Handbook of Speech Pathology* (ed. by L. E. Travis). New York: Appleton-Century Crofts, 313–388.

Hardy, William G. 1961. "Auditory Deficits of the Kernicterus Child." *Kernicterus and Its Importance in Cerebral Palsy* (ed. by C. A. Swinyard). Springfield: Charles C. Thomas, 255–266.

Harris, G. G. 1963. "Periodicity Perception by Using Gated Noise." *J. Acoustical Soc. Am.*, **35**:1229–1233.

Haymaker, W., A. Pentscew, R. Lindenberg and O. Stockdorph. 1961. "Pathology of Kernicterics and Posticteric Encephalopathy," *Kernic-*

terus and Its Importance in Cerebral Palsy (ed. by C. A. Swinyard). Springfield: Charles C Thomas, 21–230.

Jerger, James. 1957. "Auditory Adaptation." *J. Acoustical Soc. Am.,* **29**:357–363.

Katsuki, Y., N. Suga and Y. Kanno. 1962. "Neural Mechanism of the Peripheral and Central Auditory System in Monkeys." *J. Acoustical Soc. Am.,* **34**:1396–1410.

Kelemen, G. 1956. "Erythroblastosis Fetalis. Pathologic Report on the Hearing Organs of a Newborn Infant." *Arch. Otol.,* **63**:392–398.

Kiang, N. Y.-S., T. Watanabe, E. C. Thomas and L. F. Clark. 1962. "Stimulus Coding in the Cat's Auditory Nerve." *Tr. Am. Otol. Soc.,* **50**:264–281.

Kiang, N. Y.-S., R. R. Pfeiffer, W. B. Warr and A. S. N. Backus. 1965. "Stimulus Coding in the Cochlear Nucleus." *Tr. Am. Otol. Soc.,* **53**:35–57.

Licklider, J. C. R. 1959. "Three Auditory Theories." *Psychology: A Study of a Science* (ed. by S. Koch). New York: McGraw-Hill, **1**:41–145.

Licklider, J. C. R. 1962. "Periodicity Pitch and Related Auditory Process Models." *Internat. Audiology,* **1**:11–36.

Malamud, N. 1961. "Pathogenesis of Kernicterus in the Light of its Sequelae." *Kernicterus and Its Importance in Cerebral Palsy* (ed. by C. A. Swinyard). Springfield: Charles C. Thomas, 230–244.

Matkin, N. D. 1965. "Audiological Patterns Characterizing Hearing Impairments Due to Rh Incompatibility." Ph.D. dissertation. Northwestern University.

Miller, G. A. and W. C. Taylor. 1948. "The Perception of Repeated Bursts of Noise." *J. Acoustical Soc. Am.,* **20**:171–182.

Newby, H. A. 1964. *Audiology,* 2nd ed. New York: Appleton-Century Crofts.

Nieder, P. C. and C. D. Creelman. 1965. "Central Periodic Pitch." *J. Acoustical Soc. Am.,* **37**:136–138.

Perlstein, M. A. 1961. "The Clinical Syndrome of Kernicterus." *Kernicterus and Its Importance in Cerebral Palsy* (ed. by C. A. Swinyard). Springfield: Charles C. Thomas, 268–279.

Ritsma, R. J. 1962. "Existence Region of the Total Residue I." *J. Acoustical Soc. Am.,* **34**:1224–1229.

Rose, J. 1960. "Organization of Frequency Sensitive Neurons in the Cochlear Nucleus Complex of the Cat." *Neural Mechanisms of the*

Auditory Vestibular Systems (ed. by G. Rasmussen and W. E. Windle). Springfield: Charles C. Thomas, 116–136.

Rosen, J. 1956. "Variations in the Auditory Disorders of the Rh Child." *J. Speech & Hearing Disorders*, **21**:418–422.

Schouten, J. F. 1962. "The Residue Phenomenon and its Impact on the Theory of Hearing." *Internat. Audiology*, **1**:7–10.

Small, A. M., Jr. and R. A. Campbell. 1961. "Masking of Pulsed Tones by Bands of Noise." *J. Acoustical Soc. Am.*, **33**:1570–1576.

Tasaki, I. 1960. "Afferent Impulses in Auditory Nerve Fibers and the Mechanism of Impulse Initiating in the Cochlea." *Neural Mechanisms of the Auditory and Vestibular Systems* (ed. by G. Rasmussen and W. E. Windle). Springfield: Charles C. Thomas, 40–47.

Thompson, G. 1963. "A Modified SISI Technique for Selected Cases with Suspected Acoustic Neurinoma." *J. Speech & Hearing Disorders*, **28**:299–302.

Thurlow, W. R. and A. M. Small, Jr. 1955. "Pitch Perception for Certain Periodic Auditory Stimuli." *J. Acoustical Soc. Am.*, **27**:132–137.

Wever, Glen. 1949. *Theory of Hearing.* New York: John Wiley and Sons.

GEORGE E. SHAMBAUGH, JR.

DISCUSSION: MEDICAL TREATMENT AND RESEARCH

CONSIDERING the contributions of Drs. Goodhill and Carhart on kernicterus deafness, I find it remarkable how short a time it is since this was first thought of and recognized and how much has been learned. Yet we still do not know the final answer. As Dr. Goodhill has emphasized, there are not yet adequate studies of the temporal bones, the central nervous system and audiometric tests on any of these cases. Dr. Carhart has given us the fascinating deductive reasoning that the lesions are in the cochlear nuclei in the brain stem, but I don't think we can finally conclude that this is the whole story until pathologic evidence is complete. I was intrigued by Dr. Goodhill's comment that the day of Rh deafness, kernicteric deafness, is drawing to a close with the transfusion of the fetus in the 30th day of pregnancy, if I am not mistaken. I'm rather intrigued as to how this could be done.

Dr. Guilford emphasized one of my pet subjects: the importance of allergy in secretory otitis media in childhood, and secretory otitis media in childhood is an important medical situation that we can do something about. These cases are very common. They seem to be increasing in frequency, or else we are becoming more keen in recognizing them. And we must remember that patients with severe sensorineural losses are not at all immune to a superimposed secretory otitis. These cases are very easily overlooked. We must keep our eyes open and remain aware of the fact that treatment of the secretory otitis in such a child can give him a

252

very useful improvement in hearing, although of course not normal hearing. Fortunately, most of these allergic children are allergic to house dust, at least in Chicago, and they respond very well to what we call the optimum dosage method of treatment. I'm calling to my mate now, because those of you who are not doctors will not know what I'm talking about. But the fact remains they respond very well to treatment. Some of them require polyethylene tube insert; others require an adenoidectomy, but most of them can be brought under control.

The problem of surgery for congenital malformations is an interesting one, and I agree that these cases are not so very common. There was a very disturbing report a few years ago from Philadelphia in which this otologist claimed that these congenital malformations were contributing to many children with severe sensorineural losses and could be benefited through surgery. I don't want to mention his name because I think it was a very bad report. In the first place he said that in every case he had operated he had found something wrong. Then he described what he found wrong, which I think coincides with the normal anatomical variations we see when we open up the middle ear. Secondly, he was unable to confirm the fact that these children had better hearing for conversation after his operations. He said that he was only able to demonstrate improvement by EDA testing. At least, that was my conclusion from his paper. In other words, the usual speech and pure-tone testing did not show improvement, so I'm very doubtful that he really had improvements in these cases. I think this was a bad paper because it arouses so much false hope amongst the parents of these deaf children. As Dr. Lowell emphasized, and this is extremely important, the parents of the deaf child resist for weeks, months and sometimes years the acceptance of the fact that their child is deaf and has an irreversible deafness, and they will grasp at a straw time and again. It is very unfortunate when something of this sort gets into the lay press, because these parents once again have their hopes aroused and will rush off to the next person who has something they think to offer them rather than concentrating on the problem at hand. Amongst the miracle cures, of course, which we read about in the press in the past four or five years, is that of the electronic implant to stimulate directly the auditory nerve. And this, of course, aroused tremendous hopes in the parents of deaf children. Of course, they were vain hopes. In the July 1966 issue of the *Archives of Otolaryngology* there appeared a very interesting report on the electric implant—pessimistic as to its eventual value, but very interesting.

Just when is surgery indicated in these deaf children? First of all, if they have a secretory otitis media this must be controlled. Some of them require adenoidectomy—this is a form of surgery; some require polyethylene tube placed through the tympanic membrane. This is a minor form of surgery. Those who go on to develop a cholesteatoma, and some of these do, as Dr. Guilford demonstrated, must have surgery, because this is a bone-invading process which if neglected becomes worse inevitably and eventually threatens life. Some children have a congenital cholesteatoma. This too is a bone-invading process wherein surgery is mandatory.

On the other hand, in cases of congenital malformation, including atresia of the ear, we do not need to rush into surgery. These children do well with hearing aids, and there is an advantage in waiting until the child is older. In the first place, the growth of the bones of the ear is completed, so that surgery can be better accomplished. In the second place, we can do the surgery under local anesthesia if the child is 14 or 15 or 16 years old, and the surgeon can do a better job than under general anesthesia. Thirdly our diagnostic tests are much more reliable as the child grows older. And so I think there is little indication for rushing into surgery on these congenital malformations— positive or suspected. It is better to wait, if in doubt.

Now, nobody likes to talk about his bad results, but I would like to present two examples to emphasize some of these points. The first one is a patient who came to me at the age of 12 with a severe hearing loss. There seemed to be an air-bone gap, and this seemed to be borne out not only in the audiogram but in the tuning-fork tests (Figure 1). It was, however, for the low frequencies up to 1000 but not beyond. It was not a large air-bone gap and I was not certain at all that this was a surgically correctible defect, but I felt that exploration was justified on the poorer ear. But I call your attention to the discrimination score in the left ear, the poorer ear—only 18 percent. The next audiogram shows the result after surgery, five years later (Figure 2). We had brought the poorer ear up to where the pure tones are a trifle better than the good ear but the discrimination is no good at all in that ear. This operation was of no value to the patient. This was one of

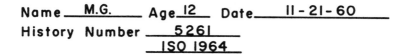

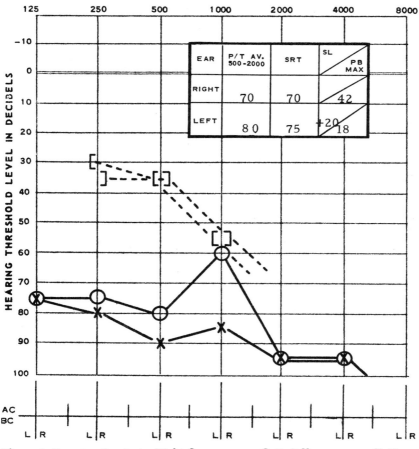

Figure 1. Preoperative tests. Right **O————O. Left X————X.** Bone dotted.

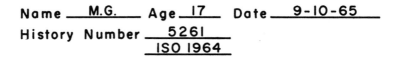

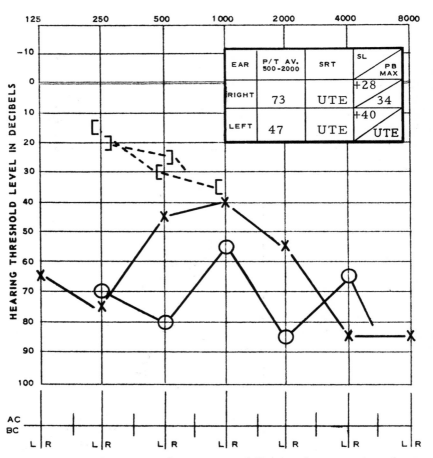

Figure 2. Tests five years after stapes mobilization for correction of conductive deficit left ear.

these cases with a profuse perilymph escape which often is harmful to the inner ear, and I would consider this as an unsuccessful operation, although the pure tones do show some improvement.

The next example is a less happy case. This is a child who came to me from St. Louis. I think Dr. Goldstein examined this child previously and there seemed to be a genuine air-bone gap for those low frequencies. I was encouraged or urged by the parents to explore this patient. I tried to give them a very limited prognosis. X-Ray studies did show what appeared to be a bony bridge between the malleus and the wall of the middle ear. I told them it looked as though part of his loss might be conductive and that by removing this conductive deficit we might get some improvement, but that he would remain a very hard of hearing child (Figure 3). Notice that his discrimination was not obtainable in either ear before surgery. The parents were most eager to have this child operated. In fact, psychologically, this was a child who already had been thoroughly rejected by his mother. I was told by the nurse in my office who took the history that if the operation did not succeed she thought the mother would probably push the child out the window. I am on the 37th floor, so this would have been very final. At any rate, I explored the child, and I found absolutely nothing abnormal. The ossicles were perfectly mobile, there was no bony bridge such as the X-Ray had suggested, and, of course, no hearing improvement. And the parents are even more unhappy than before (Figure 4). This patient would be much better off had he not been operated. I think we must be very guarded about interpreting hearing tests in these very deaf children who seem to show an air-bone gap for the low frequencies, and I think the longer we can wait before we explore these children probably the better, until we can get more reliable hearing tests when the child is older.

I should like to make one concluding comment. We have been presented with a few brief, not too fierce arguments as to whether the otologist, the pediatrician, or the audiologist should carry the ball on these deaf children. Well, I think the answer is pretty obvious. In the first place, the pediatrician first sees the child, and the pediatrician must have a high index of suspicion and must know enough about the rudimentary testing of hearing of infants that they can at least suspect the cases which should have further investigation. Then the otologist must see these

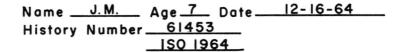

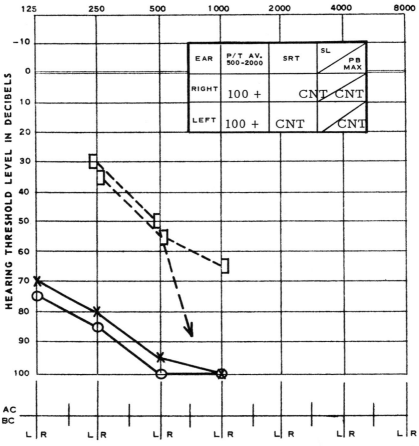

Figure 3. Preoperative tests, second case. Right O————O. Left X————X. Bone dotted.

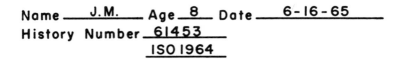

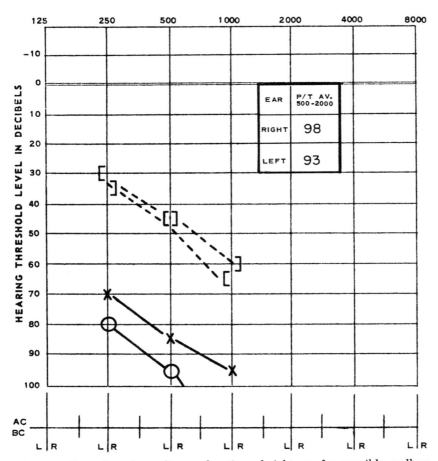

Figure 4. Tests five days after exploration of right ear for possible malleus fixation, not present.

patients, because some of them do have a definite medical situation which can be improved by treatment; and eventually some of them do have a severe conductive deficit which can be restored. The direction of the education of these children is, however, the big problem, and this must be under the guidance of someone with the time to do it. The otologist doesn't; neither does the pediatrician. It must be the audiologist.

Dr. Brown's chapter is most interesting, but I'm afraid my knowledge of genetics is not sufficient to add anything very important to it. I was encouraged by the fact that two deaf parents could expect to have 60 percent normal hearing children. This to me is rather amazing. I still would not encourage two deaf people to marry if they are congenitally deaf.

PART **V**

**AUDIOLOGIC
AND EDUCATIONAL
TREATMENT
AND RESEARCH**

CHAPTER **16** LEO CONNOR

RECENT TRENDS IN EDUCATION
OF THE DEAF

THE education of deaf children is an area of special education. Special education's ultimate objective is the eradication of the effects of any handicapping conditions which could not be prevented, while its practical goal is to provide to handicapped children the best education possible without regard to expense, convenience, or educational practices. Special education is an integral part of the field of education. It is a social science. Special educators, therefore, are practical social scientists dedicated to the influencing of human behavior through the teaching-learning process and the utilization of the knowledge, skills and materials provided by any other professional, technical, or applied area of human activity.

Special Education's major and unique aim is the developmental instruction of handicapped children, from the youngest to the oldest, in the educational skills, knowledge, and attitudes that are deemed vital to the independent adult living of individuals in modern society.

Educators of the deaf are a professional group who have as their main objective the instruction of deaf children of all ages, of all varieties of hearing impairment, in all settings, with all methods and materials, in all areas of the curriculum and under the direction of educational personnel.

The education of the deaf is one of the smaller divisions of the field of education. As illustrated in Figure 1, it is an eclectic instructional field that reaches out to the best and the newest in

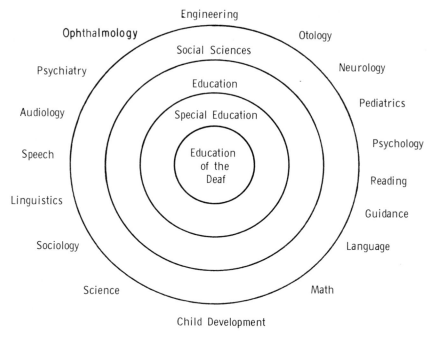

Figure 1. The relation of education of the deaf to other fields.

various fields to augment its purposes. It rests upon the finding of neurologists, of pediatricians, of otologists, of ophthalmologists, and of psychiatrists. It culls from the findings of audiologists, of speech clinicians, of linguistic scientists, of sociologists, of anthropologists, of psychologists, and of child-development specialists. It utilizes the newest creations of various engineering fields, of electronic activities, of computer and data retrieval enterprises, and of the television and audio-visual fields. Finally, it calls upon the experts in each curriculum area, including speech, auditory training, speechreading, language, social studies, mathematics, reading, guidance, vocational subjects, and science. In short, it feeds upon the content, methodology, and the skills of every liberal and applied art. Its finished product is an independent, mature deaf young man or woman able to accept and be accepted in the world of the nonhandicapped. Any less ideal is failure.

Education must lay claim to the deaf child during the first year of life. Although medical diagnosis may be incomplete, the existence of any of the following "high-risk" indicators would suggest frequent attention by the education specialist to insure vital assistance as an early age in the development of language: babies born of congenitally deaf parents; babies born of mothers with certain first trimester pregnancy symptoms; babies who have suffered attacks of meningitis, high fever or viral infections; and babies found to have discernible hearing losses.

Several centers throughout the United States are following the example of those in England, Japan, and the Scandanavian countries, where baby and parent training are accepted procedures. The Tracy Clinic, the Central Institute for the Deaf, the Atlanta Speech School, the Lexington School for the Deaf, and the Bill Wilkerson Center have inagurated educational services for these youngest of hearing-impaired subjects. Their programs usually include parental guidance and instruction, as well as speech, language, and auditory training instruction for the child. The instruction is individually geared to the unfolding diagnostic picture and probably will be responsible for much of the needed diagnostic information and prognostic estimates.

In addition, home teaching by a teacher of the deaf is a growing, vital aspect of the educational process. It involves the systematic concentration upon all sensory avenues of language and speech input starting in the crib and should add the support of counseling and psychological services for the parents of hearing impaired babies.

Nursery education for the deaf child with its emphasis upon the gamut of emotional, social, physical, and intellectual development of three- and four-year-old children has never been national in practice within this country. Although nursery education was initiated for deaf children during the 1930s, it is estimated that fewer than half of the deaf children in the United States receive daily nursery instruction. Deaf children must be started in educational pursuits earlier; they must be kept at it longer and they must work harder. The single major need for any deaf child is for a consistent overwhelming quantity of straight language input and output.

The method of instruction at this age is one of concentrated individual tutoring surrounded by the best of nursery activities to foster general areas of human development. Deaf children cannot be satisfied with once-a-week clinical speech or language instruction. Parents and professional groups interested in the fullest development of the deaf child undoubtedly will demand that daily, full-day nursery programs be available from education agencies to provide intensive activities with qualified personnel. The aim for every deaf child is to initiate and establish habitual speech-reading, understandably articulated speech, and a receptive and expressive vocabulary of hundreds of words and verbal concepts by the fifth birthday.

Whether the deaf child ever did or can "think without language" is a useless question to debate, for the deaf child *must* think *with* language like every other human being. The total immersion of the deaf child into language as early as possible and the deaf child's command of all areas of the language arts activities are ideal educational goals for him. It seems unreasonable ever to expect the average deaf child to overcome fully his profound handicap, but education must accept that goal as its major focus of activity to be achieved to the fullest extent possible.

Language investigations in this country and elsewhere are opening up new areas of knowledge and practical applications. Cooper and Rosenstein (1966) have stated that investigators of children's language have begun to abandon the nonlinguistic approach employed in most of the psychological studies reported before the mid–1950s. The newer investigations describe children's language at various stages in terms of their acquired grammar. Contemporary learning theory is relevant here, since discrimination learning could help the deaf learner to differentiate appropriate skills and information while discovery methods might emphasize active efforts of the learner rather than passive participation. Ideas related to programmed instruction, such as task-analysis, the specification of instructional objectives in behavioral terms, and the individualization of instruction, can provide clues to improved curriculum results in all areas of school learning. The techniques of operant conditioning also have interesting implications for the reinforcement and fixation of desirable language habits.

DiCarlo (1964) has indicated that, in the absence of audition, the teaching of speech must convey to the deaf child some concept of how speech sounds are produced; he must articulate them in sequential units; he needs precise graphic symbols for each speech sound, and he needs an environment of oral expectation and assistance.

Current trends in this area include sonographic analysis of speech production for information concerning developmental articulations under controlled conditions of input and output, as well as visible speech or graphic representations of speech production that can provide direct and consistent feedback to the deaf speaker. Auditory and tactile aids for the teaching of speech and development of audition skills are also receiving concentrated attention in many European, Canadian, and American centers. Frisina (1966) has estimated that 30 to 40 percent of pupils in schools and classes for the deaf are hard of hearing, another 30 to 40 percent classified as deaf can benefit substantially from the use of their residual hearing, and the remainder are in the "deaf-deaf" category for whom current audiological and physiological research have not provided effective assistance through the ear. Filtering and transposition of frequencies as well as low-frequency gains for hearing aids, however, offer hope of immediate, effective assistance for more and more children in the deafest group.

Advances in curriculum development and revisions of traditional curricular content are areas of general educational activity that are infusing a few school programs for the deaf with auto-instruction and intensive analysis of subject-matter content. Starting after the impact of "sputnik," the field of education inaugurated sweeping revisions of content and methodology. "New math" is probably the best known of the curriculum changes with its concentration upon the discovery of mathematical processes, the consistency of arithmetic principles, and the early introduction of higher mathematical concepts. All of the areas of science have been revised, however, with a "new biology," a "new chemistry" and a "new physics." These are available to those few schools for the deaf in the United States that offer a worthy secondary program. Linguistic approaches to the teaching of English are another manifestation of the current upsurge. Several schools of thought, ranging from generative transformational grammars to a Tagmemic approach and the Initial Teaching Alphabet, are competing for attention and trial in programs for deaf children and may even be in use in several experimental centers. Table I list a number of the current innovations that have been introduced in various schools and centers.

The fields of education in general and the education of the deaf in particular seem to be entering a scientific phase that stresses the evaluative and technological aspects of the teaching-learning process. Large sums of money, available for the first

TABLE I

CURRICULUM INNOVATIONS (EDUCATION OF THE DEAF)

Pre-Nursery:	Speech:
Home Teaching	Sonograph Analysis
Parental Counseling	Visible Speech Approaches
Tutoring (Speechreading, etc.)	Tactile Aids
	Filtering of Frequencies
	Transposition of Frequencies
Language:	**Curriculum:**
Task Analysis	New Math, New Physics, etc.
Auto-Instruction	Audio-Visual Aids
Operant Conditioning	Computer and Data Retrieval
Generative Transformational	Programmed Instruction
Grammar	Educational Research
Tagmemic Linguistics	
Initial Teaching Alphabet	

time from federal sources, have brought within reach research and experiments which utilize expensive machines, national testing, and sampling procedures, the computer and informational retrieval approaches, as well as audiovisual, closed-circuit television and programmed instruction developments. Libraries are now broadly defined as curriculum centers. The usual goal of students is becoming the completion of college and graduate study. Operation Head Start indicates that deprived children will benefit from starting school two years before the previously accepted age, and the challenges of automation are manifest in the establishment of the National Technical Institute for the Deaf and regional educational research and development centers.

Increased attention is being paid to individualized instruction of deaf pupils. The prime mover in this direction was the initiation of programmed instruction, but it has been hastened by other technological developments, notably closed-circuit television, video tape, 8mm films and computer usage. Although teachers of the deaf in general may dislike "losing classroom time" by turning to programmed instruction, some innovators find it helpful to provide interesting and meaningful drill; to provide small group or individual instruction while the larger group is occupied with the teacher; and to remedy gaps in the class instruction or to pinpoint existing areas of deficiency. The greatest learning that can be attained in this area occurs when teachers discover that they need a thorough knowledge of their subject in order to program it for pupils.

Beyond these obvious effects on the usual educational process lies the realization that the new technological devices allow teachers to move closer to the goal of specifying an individual instructional regime for multiply handicapped deaf children. The pace and the sequence of content can thus be independently controlled for each student based upon his responses to the material. Teachers of the future will spend more time in programming significant parts of their lessons, in diagnosing pupil learning problems, and in remedying them in close tutorial interactions. A nongraded, continuous-progress plan with independent tracks then will become possible for the deaf students with additional problems which are causing so much current professional distress.

Educational research in the United States concerned with the deaf has increased gradually within the past ten years as the result of a few interested individuals and under the stimulation of federal governmental programs. The majority of the professional researchers responsible for this progress have been from the fields of psychology, medicine, and audiology. Despite a few notable gains and even more exciting prospects, it is still true that the present quantity and quality of research in the education of deaf children remains disappointingly low, and its application in the instructional realm is almost nonexistent.

The major research trends currently seem to be revolving around the areas of language, concept formation and levels of thinking, acoustical processes, programmed learning, neurological impairment, and differential diagnosis. Many gaps exist, indicating the lack of large-scale investigations into such areas as methodology; child development norms; parental and community attitudes; administrative and teacher effectiveness; standardized instruments for diagnosis, achievement and prediction; perceptual and neurological processes involved in the classroom; social and vocational development; and experimental teaching devices and environmental influences.

The variety of educational research techniques must be widened. Historical and experimental studies should be strengthened while the descriptive and retrospective research now available is continued. Longitudinal data are required on larger numbers of deaf children to check the overgeneralized results usually reported after analysis of small group, cross-sectional, geographically restricted data obtained from studies now conducted in this country.

The greatest need in the area of research that deaf children have is for classroom practices to be improved by the vast amount of educational research findings now available in the journals, textbooks, and library shelves of this country. Educators cannot afford to live on the reputation of work done in other fields or on piecemeal approaches to the problems of skills, methods, terminology, learning, objectives, personnel, attitudes, and curriculum that affect deaf children.

The professional preparation of personnel to work in educational programs with deaf children is entering a new era of specialization. As widespread research efforts expand the kinds of knowledge available, older personnel must be "retreaded" while present preparation programs will become more rigorous and extensive (Quigley, 1966). The specialization will require different preparation programs for teachers of nursery and kindergarten deaf children, while secondary teachers should be certified in their content areas as well as in the education of the deaf. Supervisors and principals no longer can be promoted out of the classroom without the completion of specific graduate training, internships in these leadership positions, and the updating and broadening of their content information.

The reorientation of the professional preparation process indicts the conception of an *ad hoc* set of successful recipes in the framework of a definite course of action (Coladorci, 1956). Such a strategy seems to be at the root of much of the current dissatisfaction with beginning teachers (Coulson, 1966), since no system that sets up certain teacher personality characteristics or blocks of subject matter to be mastered can mandate for the combination of variables emanating from the classroom, the community, and the faculty. Rather, a new approach indicates that the educational act is an uninterrupted cycle of inquiry, beginning with educated hypotheses based on information as to what methods, materials and professional behavior are likely to bring about the desired criterial changes. The effectiveness of these hypotheses as manifested in the classroom will then be tested and reinforced or modified by objective evaluations. Teacher preparation programs must begin to provide the relevant theoretical, technical, and behavioral experiences necessary for intelligent hypothesizing and their testing in the reality of a classroom.

Another approach along similar lines is the concept of the diagnostic (Connor, 1959) or prescriptive (Peter, 1965) teacher. Thus, classroom decisions arise when there is a discrepancy between the actual behavior of a pupil and the behavior that the teacher wants the child to have.The teacher has three tasks: the diagnosis of pupil difficulty, the setting up of goals and incentives; and the choice of remedial or developmental procedures.

It is therefore proposed that the professional preparation of teachers stress the initial assessment of pupil status to the extent that specific pupil problems are isolated, his errors en route to desirable behavior examined, and then a choice of remedial measures provided to assist his own self-learning activity.

In conclusion, the education of the deaf child has been benefitting and will continue to benefit even more from the surge of attention, research, dissatisfactions, financial investments, and international communication available in the 1960s. The United States Department of Health, Education and Welfare (Advisory Committee on the Education of the Deaf, 1965) has, after a national study, concluded that a massive, countrywide effort must be made over the next five years substantially to upgrade the traditionally accepted language arts deficiencies of the deaf. If such efforts are not bogged down by the Viet Nam war, political expediencies, or the power plays of the educational establishment among our school administrators, then the new attitudes that question and defy so-called "accepted" facts hold promise of some exciting vistas for the future in the education of deaf children.

References

Advisory Committee on the Education of the Deaf. 1965. "Education of the Deaf." *A Report to the Secretary of Health, Education, and Welfare on the Education of the Deaf.* U. S. Department of Health, Education and Welfare. Washington, D. C.: U. S. Government Printing Office.

Coladorci, A. P. 1956. "The Relevancy of Educational Psychology." *Educational Leadership,* **13**:489–492.

Connor, Leo E. 1959. "Diagnostic Teaching." *Volta Review,* **61**:311–314.

Cooper, Robert and Joseph Rosenstein. 1966. "Language Acquisition of Deaf Children." *Volta Review,* **68**:58–67.

Coulson, J. E. 1966. "Automation, Electronic Computers, and Education." *Phi Delta Kappa,* **47**:340–344.

DiCarlo, Louis. 1964. *The Deaf.* Englewood Cliffs, New Jersey: Prentice-Hall, Inc.

Frisina, D. R. 1966. Speech at University of Nebraska Symposium on Systems Approach to the Education of the Deaf, April 1966. University of Nebraska Press (in press).

Peter, L. J. 1965. *Prescriptive Teaching.* New York: McGraw-Hill.

Quigley, Steven (ed.). 1966. *Preparation of Teachers of the Deaf.* U. S. Office of Education. Washington, D. C.: U. S. Government Printing Office.

PSYCHOEDUCATIONAL MANAGEMENT OF THE YOUNG DEAF CHILD

THE definition of schizophrenia refers to a division, or splitting, of the personality. It may be that a little schizophrenia will be helpful in considering my topic, "Psychoeducational Management of the Young Deaf Child." Although we are primarily concerned with the young deaf child and the special set of needs that his sensory deficit creates, we must split off another major part of our attention for the parents of these children. For parents are the key to successful psychoeducational management.

In considering the role that parents play in successful psychoeducational management, it is possible to distinguish a number of stages. We have labeled these stages awareness, acceptance, information, and application.

We want first to become aware of the possibility of a hearing loss at the earliest possible time. The recent International Meeting in Toronto on the problems of early detection of hearing loss was an indication of the great interest in this subject and highlighted the progress that is being made in many countries through infant screening programs, the registration and follow-up of all children born at-risk, and improved techniques for both behavioral and physiological measurements of hearing in infancy. In fact, the paper by Wedenburg (1964), presented at Toronto on prenatal testing, would seem to be carrying early detection about as far as one would care to go.

We are also concerned with increasing public awareness of the possibility of early deafness. We must do what we can to help create in parents an awareness that deafness may be the reason their child's behavior is different.

A number of professions are important in creating early awareness—the pediatrician, the otologist, and the audiologist are all involved. In a study of 1,500 young deaf children enrolled in our correspondence course (Lowell *et al.*, 1957), we found that medical personnel were responsible for approximately 40 percent of the initial determinations of loss, while audiologists accounted for another 48 percent of the initial determinations. It is clear that this is a shared responsibility.

One influence we have to fight is what might be called the "don't-be-a-neurotic-mother syndrome." Under the benign Spockian influence, we still find mothers who are told, "Now don't worry. It may just be fluid in his ears"; or, "Bring him back when he is older and we can test him." The increased availability of the pediatric-otologic-audiologic team is doing much to overcome this problem.

The second stage in the psychoeducational management of the young deaf child is acceptance. Detection is only half of the battle if the parents are unwilling, or unable, to accept the fact that their child is deaf. Parents frequently need help in accepting that fact fully and emotionally.

Very few parents have had any experience with deafness, let alone with young deaf children. For them, the specter of the unknown does as much as anything else to retard acceptance. It helps to have them see other deaf children playing and learning. At John Tracy Clinic, we find that talking with other parents of deaf children—parents who share the same concerns and anxieties and who have had the same questions—helps parents in the emotional acceptance of the fact of deafness.

Despite all our efforts, it is understandable that, just beneath the surface, all parents of deaf children have a very active and compelling hope that the tests may be wrong, that the hearing will improve, that some new medical discovery will be made tomorrow. The best evidence we have of the strength of this hope is the great amount of mail that reaches our Clinic every time some new miracle operation or cure is reported in the public press. The last major report of this sort brought us letters from literally all over the world, from parents who were ready to bring their child to Southern California to be operated on.

The first person to confront the parents with the diagnosis of

education has for language acquisition. We estimate that the av-
deafness plays an important part in helping them to accept it. If
he is equivocal in his decision, if he holds out false hope, he
may be doing the parents a great disservice.

The next step after detection and acceptance is to provide the
parents with information. They need a great deal of information
about the role that they can play in their child's education, about
the acquisition of language, speech, the use of hearing aids, auditory training—in fact, all of the areas that contribute to a deaf
child's education. The acquisition of language by hearing people
is as yet imperfectly understood. This makes our task of com-
municating the little that is known to parents even more challenging.

Parents initially think only in terms of, "Will my child speak?"
while the educator's concern is with the acquistion of language.
It takes time to convince parents that language must come first,
and that they must fill the reservoir of receptive language before
they begin to see even the beginnings of consistent meaningful
speech.

There is a growing contribution to this pool of information
about the importance of early education. I am thinking particularly of a paper by Penfield (1964) on "The Uncommitted Cortex," which substantiates neurologically what teachers of the
deaf have been telling parents about the critical language-learn-
ing years. Linguists inform us that, in children with normal hearing, the acquisition of grammatical structure of the language is
virtually complete by three and one half to four years of age.
We must see that parents understand the implications and are
motivated to act accordingly.

We are beginning to see a great contribution from instructional
technology in getting this information across to parents. Programmed and automated instruction, video tapes, films, slides,
and recordings can be a great asset, particularly when we attempt
to teach parents of different intellectual levels and educational
backgrounds the many facts that will help them to function effectively in their child's education.

The final step is application. Awareness, acceptance, and information go for naught if parents are unable to address themselves to the important task of guiding their child's learning.
Time is of the essence here, and I wonder how often we think of
the amount of time that a child who requires primarily visual

erage preschooler sleeps about ten hours at night, and with another hour out for a nap, he has thirteen hours of waking time. Of this, at least half is spent in activities that require the child's eyes for other purposes, which leaves only six and one half hours a day available for the acquisition of language through the eyes. Not only do we have a deficient sensory input, but we have not even comparable time for that less efficient sensory channel to operate. It is clear that parents must make maximum use of all the available time.

I wonder how many medical men realize how important they are in insuring application. The doctor who stresses the importance of education to the parents, who tells them, "This is what you must do," almost in the form of a prescription, is a great asset to the educator. For parents who have recently learned of their child's deafness, this is probably the single most effective motivator that we have. It is the one prescription that will insure application.

We are also beginning to see new and very exciting forms of application. At our own Clinic (U.S. Office of Education, 1965) and at the Bill Wilkerson Center in Nashville, as well as at several other centers throughout the United States, we are experimenting with a new format for presenting information to parents. Rather than teaching parents in a classroom or clinic what they should do at home, we are now teaching them in a simulated home, where routine household activities are used as the vehicle for the teaching. Parents, with skillful guidance and direction, are shown the many opportunities available for language learning in everyday activities and how to make maximum use of them. We believe that teaching in a home-like setting will increase the likelihood of transfer and application in the real home. It is a concept that I am sure we will see emulated in many other localities throughout the United States.

In summary, what can we say about the results of our attempts at psychoeducational management? The information that we have is not very encouraging. Pintner and Reamer (1920) studied 2,000 children in schools for the deaf. Their conclusions were that deaf children were approximately two years behind hearing children of the same age on intelligence tests and five years behind them educationally.

Some 45 years later, a report by the Secretary of Health, Education, and Welfare's Advisory Committee on the Education of the Deaf (1965) showed that "The average graduate of a public residential school for the deaf—the closest we have to generally available high schools for the deaf—has an eighth-grade education." It would appear that we have not made much progress in 45 years.

All educators hope that we could somehow close this gap so that the deaf student upon entering the world of work would be as well prepared as a hearing person. Where are we to look for the time and the opportunity? I doubt that we will do much catching up through improved teaching methods—the application of technology, for example—for as these techniques are applied to the deaf, they will also be applied to hearing children, so that the gap between them will be maintained.

There are, however, two areas which have been the most neglected and yet which seem to offer the brightest hope for improving the education of deaf children. The first would be accelerated interest in very early education, which inevitably involves the parents. From everything that has been said in this paper, it would seem reasonable to assume that greater parental involvement in the educative process, particularly at the early levels, deserves special attention. Unfortunately, our educational system is not generally equipped to offer the necessary assistance to parents or to young children, but we are seeing an increased interest in this area, and it is one in which I believe we can expect great progress.

The other area that would seem to offer considerable potential would be twelve-month schooling. I think we have already begun to work toward that goal through the growth of our summer sessions. Considering the seriousness of the problem for the deaf child, I believe it will only be a matter of time before we accept twelve-month schooling as a normal part of deaf education.

We believe that progress will be facilitated if we attend to the major variables of awareness, acceptance, information, and application. If we are able to organize our resources and bring them to bear on the problem, if we are wise enough to take advantage of the advances in technology, and if we take the time that is so essential in the psychoeducational management of the young deaf child, I believe we can be quite optimistic about the future.

References

Advisory Committee on the Education of the Deaf. 1965. "Education of the Deaf." *A Report to the Secretary of Health, Education, and Welfare.* U. S. Department of Health, Education and Welfare. U. S. Government Printing Office, Washington, D. C.

Lowell, Edgar L., Georgina Rushford, and Harriet Montague. 1957. "Survey of Families Enrolled in The John Tracy Clinic Correspondence Course." *J. Speech & Hearing Disorders,* **22**:75–86.

Penfield, Wilder. 1964. "The Uncommitted Cortex, the Child's Changing Brain." *Atlantic Monthly,* **214**:77–81.

Pintner, Rudolf, and J. F. Reamer. 1920. "A Mental and Educational Survey of Schools for the Deaf." *Am. Ann. Deaf,* **65**:451.

U. S. Office of Education. 1965. "Home Teaching for Parents of Young Deaf Children." Demonstration Project No. 32–14–0000–1014, supported by the *Division of Handicapped Children and Youth, Bureau of Educational Research and Development.*

Wedenberg, Erik. 1964. "Prenatal Tests of Hearing." *Acta-otolaryng. Suppl.,* **26**:27–30.

LEARNING WITH VISUAL AND
AUDIOVISUAL PRESENTATIONS

ONE of the aspects of deaf education on which there is fair agreement is the multisensory approach. Over the years this has taken a number of forms, but recently it has involved a combination of audition and vision plus secondary use of other modalities. The literature contains reports that the general communicative ability of the children is improved when they wear hearing aids and when auditory training is an integral part of their program, and there are suggestions of improved academic achievement. Careful search of the literature, however, fails to reveal anything very specific on the best way to incorporate auditory stimulation into the teaching process. Casual observations of young teachers might lead one to believe that auditory training is more a part of the setting-up exercises and tongue gymnastics than an integral part of the teaching of communication. One thing is clear; the literature does not contain any hard core of research that gives direction to the procedures.

At Wayne State University we have now done a number of experiments that were designed specifically to explore the audiovisual approach in deaf education. These studies were carried out primarily on children with normal hearing, but hard-of-hearing and deaf children have also been tested from day and residential schools. Our underlying hypothesis has been simple: If the use of an audiovisual presentation of communication and of material to be learned is more efficient than the presentation of the same material in either modality alone, then a task such as memorization or rote learning, which lends itself to experimental study, should provide a test of the hypothesis. On the other hand, if the audiovisual approach is beneficial only in very specific circumstances such as learning speech, then the experimental study of memorization would not be an adequate test, but the information gained should guide the teacher in how to distribute her energy.

The experimental procedure chosen was the paired-associate paradigm, using anticipation responses for part of the study and recall responses for the remainder. Stated more directly, the children were required to learn to respond with the second member of a pair whenever the first member was presented. The number of pairs varied from six to ten, and the material in the pairs included simple words, pronounceable nonsense trigrams, nonsense drawings, or novel noises. The lists of pairs for a given experiment were presented repeatedly, in different orders, auditorily, visually, or audiovisually until a certain criterion of learning was achieved. The criterion score was either the number of trials that it took a child to reach a certain level of performance or the number of correct responses made over a specified number of trials. The material was presented from magnetic tape and from visual memory drums or slide projectors. A pip on the second channel of the tape provided the synchronizing impulse to drive the memory drum or the slide projector. In the total array of experiments conducted for the main project, several thousand children have been tested who have ranged in age from about four to about eighteen or nineteen and in hearing ability from normal to totally deaf. The experiments reported here were abstracted from the group described in our final research reports released in 1960, 1963, and 1966. As just stated, the studies were designed to search for differences in performance associated with an audiovisual approach versus a visual approach alone.

The first experiment to be reported was not part of the main sequence. It was carried out as a doctoral dissertation by Graunke (1959). He utilized four groups of children. Three of the groups were from a residential school for the deaf and were classified as acoustic because they wore and utilized hearing aids, oral because they communicated through speech and lip reading, and manual because their means of communication was by finger-spelling and signing. The fourth group was made up of normal children at the fourth-grade level from the public schools. Each child learned two lists of pairs of words, one visually and another audiovisually, under conditions in which order and list effects were counter-balanced. The data revealed no differences between the two methods of presentation for the oral and manual groups. This result was expected, since all these children had very severe hearing losses and none of them was presumed to have any functional hearing. There was a significant difference in the acoustic group, only surprisingly, the audiovisual presentation was significantly poorer than the visual presentation. It was as though the addition of the auditory component had actually interfered with the performances on the task. A similar but less significant trend, however, was observed with the normal children. A careful review of the design revealed that we had overlooked the fact that the practice had been carried out visually for all children. Since it was not practical to repeat the entire experiment, a second acoustic and a second normal group were tested in which the practice was audiovisual. With the normal group the results were reversed; the audiovisual procedure was better than the visual alone. With the acoustic group, the combined presentation was still inferior but not as much as it had been initially. When the data for the two normal groups and the two acoustic groups were analyzed by means of analyses of variance, a significant interaction was found between the method of practice and the method of learning for the normal group, but for the acoustic group, the only significance that emerged was the superiority of the visual method over the combined method. These results have since been corroborated in similar experiments with improved apparatus and different groups of children.

In 1957 we began the series of experiments designed to investigate bimodal versus unimodal methods of presentation of material to be learned. In the first main experiment, nine conditions were used in which all combinations of auditory, visual, and audiovisual methods of presentation were combined in practice and in learning. Thus, for example, one of the nine groups of children practiced auditorily and learned auditorily while another group practiced visually and learned audio-visually. Of specific interest here are the three conditions in which the children practiced and learned by the three basic methods of presentation. Figure 1 presents the learning curves for three groups, thirty each, of fourth-grade children who learned the lists by the three methods of presentation. It is obvious that for this experiment there

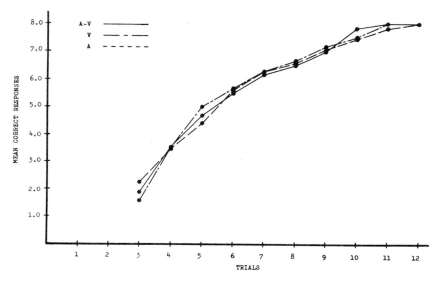

Figure 1. Learning curves for an eight word-pair list for Conditions A, V, and A–V, fourth grade.

is no difference among the three methods of presentation. The combined audiovisual method is not superior to the presentations using single modalities.

Figure 2 presents the learning curves for the same material when learned by a group of children in public schools with very mild hearing losses. For all the children in this group the average hearing level was between 16 and 30 dB, ASA 1951, for 500–2000 Hz in the better ear. In most instances, both ears were in this range, but the selection criteria specified the better ear. There were only 15 children per group, thus the curves are not as smooth as for the normal group. Again, there is no significant difference between the audiovisual procedure and the visual. The numerical difference between the two curves is slight and does not begin to approach statistical significance. Of particular interest is the fact that there is a significant deficiency in learning when the material is presented auditorily. While this is not a part of the main thesis of the presentation here, it argues for revisions in the educational management of hard-of-hearing children.

Figure 3 displays the same information from a group with average losses between 31 and 45 dB in the better ear. Again, the audiovisual approach is neither practically nor statistically su-

perior to the visual performance. Interestingly, the auditory performance from this group is at least as good as that from the

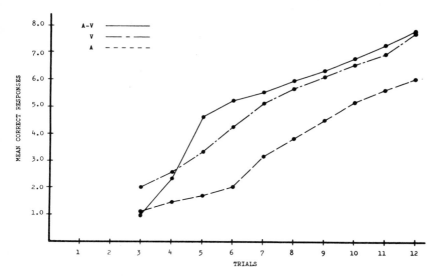

Figure 2. Learning curves for an eight word-pair list for Conditions A, V,
and A–V, 16–30 dB loss group.

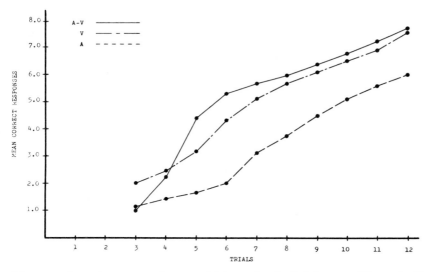

Figure 3. Learning curves for an eight word-pair list for conditions A, V,
and A–V, 31–45 dB loss group.

group with hearing losses from 16 to 30 dB. It seems possible that the two groups are in fact essentially equivalent, since the group represented by Figure 3 wore hearing aids which probably gave them aided hearing equivalent to the unaided hearing of the group with the milder hearing losses.

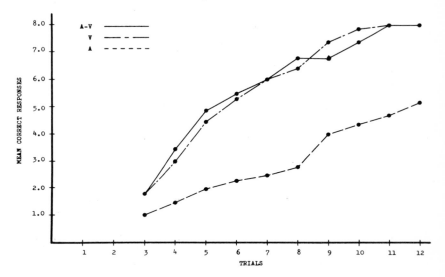

Figure 4. Learning curves for an eight word-pair list for conditions A, V, and A–V, 46–60 dB groups.

Figure 4 summarizes the results from children with hearing losses of 45 to 60 dB. The audiovisual and the visual scores are entirely equivalent, and the auditory scores are poorer than for the two preceding groups.

Figure 5 deviates from the trend. It is for a group of children with hearing losses from 61 to 75 dB. The combined procedure for this group is actually poorer than the visual procedure alone. A reasonable inference seems to be that for the groups with the milder hearing losses the auditory material was meaningful or at least intelligible to the children and thus did not interfere with the performance, although it did not help it either. In the case of the children with the hearing losses between 61 and 75 dB, the material was not very intelligible and either confused the task somewhat or distracted the children from functioning as efficiently as they did visually.

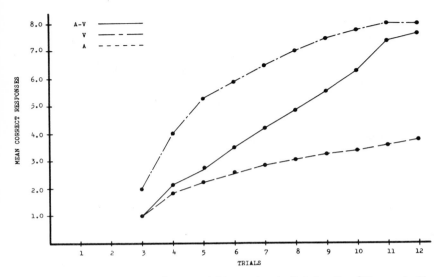

Figure 5. Learning curves for an eight word-pair list for Conditions, A, V, and A–V, 61–75 dB loss group.

The first major experiment showed repeatedly that the combined method of presentation was not superior to the visual method with hard-of-hearing children, nor superior to either the visual or the auditory with children with normal hearing. Secondarily, it highlighted the fact that hard-of-hearing children in regular schools, Figures 2, 3, and 4, were not performing auditorily as well as might have been expected from their audiograms or from their speech-discrimination scores.

In about 1960 the general format of the experiments was revised. It was reasoned that there was little basis for expecting a benefit from bimodal presentation with the simple material that had been utilized. For instance, the average school child is so familiar with the concept "dog" that the sight of the dog, the printed word "dog," the spoken word "dog," a line drawing of a dog, or even the bark of a dog are essentially equivalent in the kind of task under study. Thus, to show the printed word "dog" while someone speaks "dog" is an unnecessary redundancy. Perhaps only when the young hard-of-hearing child or the young normal child is encountering new words or new concepts is the bimodal aspect critical. The procedures and materials were redesigned, and, with the use of a slide projector, testing was carried out with groups of children rather than with the children individually. Table 1 shows the types of material utilized. Three levels of meaningfulness and/or verbalness were involved. The subscripts 1, 2, and 3 refer to the degree of meaningfulness; the capital letters refer to the sensory modality for which the stimuli were perpared or through which they could be presented. The letters in

TABLE I

STIMULUS-RESPONSE PAIRING FOR PHASE II

STIMULUS V_1	A_2 and V_2	A_3 and V_3	RESPONSE
∿	WUB	CAT	H
⊢þ	KEZ	ICE	M
∿∿	JID	ARM	V
≒	DAQ	RUG	L
⌐	WOJ	SKY	X
⌁	ZEG	GUN	F

the right column were used as responses in all instances, and the pairings were as shown in the illustration. The most meaningful and verbal materials were very simple three-letter nouns. The intermediate condition consisted of CVC trigrams that were readily pronounceable but that had been shown to be of little meaning when tested on college students (Glaze, 1928). While our earlier studies had shown that no difference was to be expected in a combined presentation of the three-letter nouns, it seemed possible that the combination of the printed material with a spoken label might make the list of nonsense syllables easier in a combined presentation than in either a visual or an auditory presentation. This combination seemed to bear reasonable similarity to the situation in which the child first sees a flash card with such a word as "cow" on it, with the teacher simultaneously speaking "cow."

V_1 items were modified from standard electric and electronic symbols. Initially, they were presented to college students who were asked to give them verbal labels or to tell what they represented or meant. The results of this work allowed us to state with some confidence that these were nonverbal and nonmeaningful symbols even though one college student thought that one of the symbols reminded him of his mother-in-law.

Because of the importance of some of the results obtained with these symbols, we later repeated one of the experiments and substituted Greek letters for this set of symbols and used other public school children. The results with the Greek letters were not different from those obtained with the symbols shown here.

Not represented in the table were six auditory "nonsense" noises. The noises were generated by manipulating and interrelating two tones that were subjected to frequency or intensity modulations and/or interruptions by electronic switches prior to being mixed and recorded. The specific manner in which they are generated is described in the original report (Gaeth, 1963).

In all, fifteen conditions were utilized with these stimuli. Each of the three lists was presented auditorily, visually, and audiovisually for a total of nine conditions. Additionally, there were six mixed conditions available, as, for instance, one in which the visual symbols were shown while the nonsense syllables were spoken, or in another, the simple nouns were spoken simultaneously with the presentation of the symbols. It seemed that the bimodal presentation of the visual symbols and the spoken nonsense syllables might result in improved performance, since the child would have a verbal label with which to manipulate the symbol. Conversely, if the noises were presented with the visual nonsense syllables, the possible associations might also be increased. Only four conditions will be used to illustrate the results.

Figure 6 presents the learning curves for the nonsense symbols and the noises. It is apparent that the visual symbols are easier to learn than the noises, but it is also obvious that the learning of the visual symbols is not improved by the inclusion of the noises. The data in this sequence of slides represent about 750 different children per slide and about 250 children per curve.

Figure 7 gives the learning curves for the three ways in which the nonsense syllables were presented. Again, the auditory presentation was not as easy as the visual presentation. There is probably a greater degree of uncertainty about these unfamiliar items when they are heard. Again, however, the combination of the auditory and visual presentation is no better than the visual presentation alone.

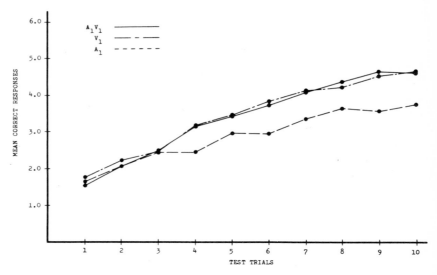

Figure 6. Learning curves for Conditions A_1, V_1, A_1V_1, grades combined.

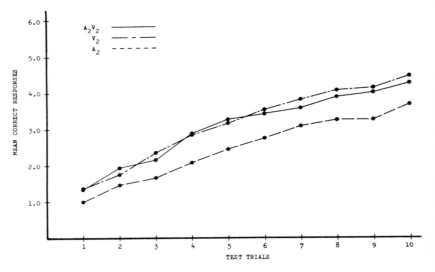

Figure 7. Learning curves for Conditions A_2, V_2, A_2V_2, grades combined.

Figure 8 is a repetition of the curve for the visual symbols and for the auditory presentation of the nonsense syllables. The combined condition of interest is one in which the nonsense syllable is spoken as the symbol is shown. If the auditory label were

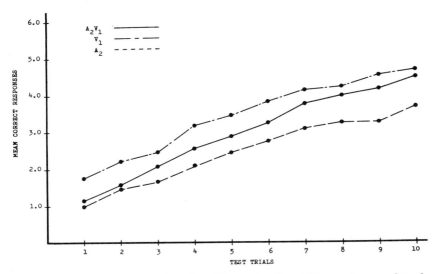

Figure 8. Learning curves for Conditions A₂, V₁, A₂V₁, grades combined.

to assist in the learning of the nonsense syllable, then the combined curve should be superior to the visual curve alone. It is interesting that the visual symbols are easier to learn than the auditory nonsense syllables, and it is even more interesting to see that the combined curve lies between the two.

Figure 9 gives the learning curves which come from the visual nonsense syllables, from the noises, and from the visual nonsense syllables being presented simultaneously with their associated noises. Again, the combined procedure does not result in improved performance.

The results shown in Figures 6–9 are typical of the results obtained from many experiments involving large numbers of children. Almost entirely without exception one can draw certain conclusions: (1) The combined auditory-visual presentation of simple words, pronounceable nonsense syllables, or nonmeaningful symbols and noises does not result in improvement of performance over single modality presentations. (2) When there is a difference in performance between the auditory and visual method of presentation, the combined presentation is never better than the better of the two unimodal presentations although it may occasionally be slightly poorer but usually not significantly so. (3) When different materials are presented via the auditory and

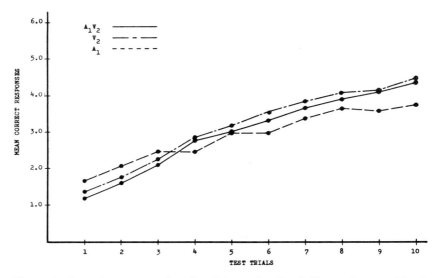

Figure 9. Learning curves for Conditions A_1, V_2, A_1V_2, grades combined.

visual channels, e.g., the visual symbols with the pronounced syllables, the performance with the combined presentation tends to be between the two individual performances when they are significantly different, or to approximate the better condition when the two unimodal conditions do not deviate markedly.

The unexpected nature of some of these findings led us to speculate on the underlying aspects of these bimodal conditions with low meaningfulness. For instance, after 10 trials with the visual symbols and the noises, an unannounced eleventh trial was introduced in which only the visual component or only the auditory component was presented to determine whether learning had taken place exclusively in one modality. The results of these experiments revealed that by the tenth trial some children were able to respond to certain items by either the visual or the auditory component separately, to items only by the visual, and for still others only by the auditory. More recently, another study was designed in which the noises and the symbols were presented in a combined task for four learning trials. At the end of the fourth trial, a test trial was given in which the six previously paired stimuli were presented as twelve separate stimuli. Thus, the letter "H" would be a correct response to the visual component as well as to the separate presentation of the auditory component. For another group of children, learning was carried on for six trials before testing was administered separately. Two other groups learned for eight and ten trials, respectively. The instructions and the learning tasks were exactly as in the other experiments until the special trial, 4, 6, 8, or 10.

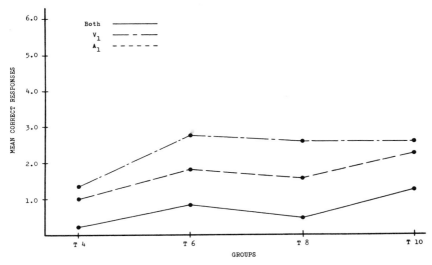

Figure 10. Mean correct responses for four trial-groups for A_1, or V_1, or both.

Figure 10 shows the mean correct responses for each of the test trials. To establish the total number of correct responses one can add the values represented for the visual and the auditory curves at each point. The score for "both" indicates the number of correct responses to both visual and auditory. Trial 6 can be used to illustrate. For this trial, on the average, the children made 2.8 correct responses to the visual stimuli and about 1.8 correct to the auditory stimuli for a total average correct of 4.6, but only about .7 correct responses to both members of the paired stimulus. The evidence here strongly suggests that initially the child learns in one modality or the other but not in both. It seems likely that the "both" represents two single learning accomplishments. In fact, the experimenters often observed children closing their eyes after about the sixth trial to see whether they could also learn the material auditorily. With normal children, the modality used to learn the material is the one which is easier for the child; normally, this is the channel containing the more meaningful material. In fact, performance can be predicted upon the basis of meaningfulness but not on the basis of sensory modality. Interestingly, the same conglomerations of experiments presented to deaf children suggest that the preceding statement must be reinterpreted, since with them the predominance of performance in the visual modality is so strong that it tends to override the more usual definition of meaningfulness. Finally, our current inference is that when individuals do show benefit from a bimodal presentation, such as in the apparent combination of lip reading and hearing through a hearing aid, it is being done, not from the integration of simultaneous bimodal presentation, but from the integration of rapidly alternating unimodal stimulation. It would appear that these data have implications for the educational management of the hard-of-hearing and deaf child.

References

Gaeth, John H. 1960. "Verbal Learning among Children with Reduced Hearing Acuity." *Final Report. Co-operative Research Project #289.* U. S. Office of Education. Department of Health, Education, and Welfare.

Gaeth, John H. 1963. "Verbal and Nonverbal Learning in Children Including Those With Hearing Losses." *Final Report, Co-operative Research Project #1001.* U. S. Office of Education. Department of Health, Education and Welfare.

Glaze, J. A. 1928. "The Associative Values of Nonsense Syllables." *J. Exp. Psychol.*, **35**:225–269.

Graunke, W. Lloyd. 1959. "Effects of Visual-Auditory Presentation on Memorization by Children with Hearing Impairments." Unpublished doctoral dissertation. Northwestern University.

CHAPTER **19** ARTHUR I. NEYHUS AND
HELMER R. MYKLEBUST

EARLY-LIFE DEAFNESS
AND MENTAL DEVELOPMENT

INVESTIGATORS in the study of the psychology of deafness
have documented the educational retardation of the deaf, beginning with the early work of Pintner (1946) and his associates.
Despite the effort put forth by educators over the decades, recent
studies continue to indicate little growth in the levels of academic achievement of those with marked deafness from birth or
from the prelanguage period (Myklebust, 1964) (Furth, 1966).
Although studies have demonstrated that the deaf child possesses
a normal level of intelligence when measured by nonverbal tests,
he has not attained the expected levels of academic learning; yet,
even with this lowered language ability, he maintains himself
independently within the community.

Research and clinical experience have indicated that the standard nonverbal intelligence tests are poor predictors of academic
achievement; it cannot be assumed that the scores achieved by
the deaf on these tests have the same meaning as for the hearing
(Birch and Birch, 1951). Only recently has attention been given
to how a deaf child learns (Furth, 1966) (Gaeth, 1964) and the
results suggest that he uses his intellectual capacity in a manner
different from that of his hearing peers. Farrant's (1964) factor-
analytic study of the intellective abilities of the deaf has
demonstrated that many of the tests employed with the hearing-
impaired factorize differently for the deaf than for the hearing;
he states further that deafness hampers the integration of mental
abilities and distorts some of them.

The basis of the adaptability of the organism is learning from experience, the root of intellectual behavior being a capacity to react to similar stimuli in a similar manner. Piaget (1960) describes this type of behavior in early life as "sensory-motor" or practical intelligence. As the child develops, his view of the world becomes intimately related to his symbolic activity. As Vigotsky (1962), Luria (1961), Werner (1963), and Bruner (1964) have postulated, mental growth occurs only as a symbol system arises, and language forms the basis for the development of human intelligence. Also, if the organism is to adapt and control its environment, a method must be available for the storage of experience.

Studies of memory among the deaf (Myklebust, 1964) (Blair, 1957) have indicated no general deficit. A qualitative difference emerges, however, when comparisons are made with the hearing. Although the deaf perform at least as well on tests concerned only with kinesthetic or visual perceptual processes and are superior on such tests as Knox Cubes and Graham-Kendall Designs, they show a marked inferiority on span test of memory, such as digits and pictures and dominoes. Whether this is related to inferior symbolic functioning must be ascertained by further research; these studies have inferred that audition has a specific effect on memory.

Contrary to the findings of the early investigators who emphasized the rigidity of thought processes, those with profound hearing losses from early life cannot be considered devoid of the capacity for abstract functioning. Oleron (1953) emphasized that the deaf have difficulty in making deductions from clues that are not observable. Although he found them to be inferior on the Raven's Progressive Matrices, Blair (1957) observed that they were capable of performing adequately on subtests of the Chicago Nonverbal Examination which require ability to conceptualize when all clues are not visible. Wright (1955) also found that Gallaudet College students were not inferior in performance on the matrices but had difficulty with items requiring arithmetical and abstract reasoning. Furth (1966) has suggested that this type of failure might be derived from experiential deficits and language incompetency, forms of cultural deprivation, rather than deficiency of abstract intelligence. He has postulated further that the deaf child is inferior in the use of logic because his method of learning has been by rote association rather than by deductive conceptualization. It is interesting to note that Templin's early studies (1950) reported that the deaf were not inferior in the use of abstract symbols but were poorer in reasoning by analogy, while the Heiders (1941) emphasized that they did not have the language tools to develop referential thinking, especially the concepts of past, future, and necessity-possibility.

The role of language in the development of thought is still being debated. For Vygotsky (1962), thought is not expressed by words but comes into existence through them. On the other hand, it appears that some types of abstract thought and behavior might not be influenced by deafness and language deficit. Yet one cannot escape the conclusion that there exists among the deaf a significant relationship between inferior development of abstraction and the verbal limitation that deafness imposes; thus, if verbal behavior is impeded, mental development may be modified reciprocally.

To gain further knowledge of the relationship between sensory defects and mental development, an investigation was made of the effects of early-life deafness on verbal acquisition and behavior. As part of a national study of the psychology of deafness, the Picture Story Test (Myklebust, 1965) was administered to more than 800 deaf children at day and residential schools. From this group, 200 stories were selected and compared with an equal number obtained from a group of hearing children matched by age, sex, and intelligence. The basic data have been reported (Myklebust, 1964), but for the purposes of this paper additional analysis has been made of the findings.

The number of different words an individual has at his command has been considered a fairly reliable index of intellectual ability (Wechsler, 1958). Table I compares the word usage of the

TABLE I

COMPARISON OF WORD USAGE BETWEEN NORMAL AND DEAF CHILDREN ON THE PICTURE STORY TEST

	Deaf					Hearing				
AGES	7	9	11	13	15	7	9	11	13	15
Number diff. words	147	260	422	512	548	162	472	556	640	1215
Total number words written	1251	1915	2100	2900	3204	769	2320	2540	3128	4535

two samples. At seven years of age, there was little difference between the groups in the number of different words employed and in the total number of words used to produce the stories. One should not draw the conclusion that the two groups are equal; rather, at this age all children have limited ability with the written word. At nine years, there was a sharp increase in the number of different words used by the hearing. The deaf children improved considerably, but they did not approach a "normal" level. At 15, there was a sharp divergence in the growth curves. The deaf had remained on a plateau since 13, while the hearing children had doubled the number of different words at their disposal. A comparison of the relative grade placements may be illustrative. The hearing youngster at 15 is in the second year of high school faced with increasing demands for skill in written language; the deaf child is in eighth grade functioning with a fifth-grade reading level. Studies of the language behavior of the adult deaf confirmed the limited verbal ability of those who have completed their education (Neyhus, 1964). Clinical experience has demonstrated that despite individual training, little significant improvement is obtained in language usage (Myklebust et al., 1962).

In terms of language usage, the 15-year-old deaf child was functioning more like the hearing child of 9 or 10, or at a ratio of three-fifths to two-thirds of average performance. This finding

TABLE II

COMPARISON OF USAGE OF PARTS OF SPEECH
BY DEAF AND HEARING CHILDREN

	Deaf Percentage of total vocabulary					Hearing Percentage of total vocabulary				
Age	7	9	11	13	15	7	9	11	13	15
Part of speech										
Noun	55.8	29.2	36.9	32.3	31.4	38.3	28.6	27.7	27.6	25.4
Verb	12.4	23.9	25.1	26.2	26.3	19.8	24.2	22.7	24.1	28.9
Adjective	18.4	16.9	15.6	16.8	14.6	12.9	13.8	17.5	14.2	16.9
Adverb	.7	6.9	6.8	7.0	5.9	7.4	10.2	6.7	10.1	9.2
Pronoun	1.4	4.2	3.3	2.9	3.9	4.3	4.5	3.8	3.9	2.6
Preposition	2.0	4.6	3.3	3.2	3.3	6.2	3.2	3.8	3.9	2.6
Conjunction	.7	1.9	1.9	1.6	1.8	1.8	1.9	1.5	4.2	1.9
Article	2.0	.8	.5	.6	.3	1.2	.4	.5	.5	.3

was similar to Myklebust's (1964) observation of the older deaf adolescents and young adults who demonstrated normal intelligence on performance tests although their verbal quotients fell at two thirds of the average. Tables II, III, and IV present further comparisons of the vocabularies of the two groups. When the frequency of usage of the various parts of speech were stud-

TABLE III

COMPARISON OF THE USE OF PARTS OF SPEECH BETWEEN
DEAF AND HEARING CHILDREN

	Deaf Percentage of total words written					Hearing Percentage of total words written				
Age	7	9	11	13	15	7	9	11	13	15
Part of speech										
Noun	43.9	31.8	33.9	26.5	26.6	28.8	26.9	24.8	22.3	18.6
Verb	17.1	20.8	16.1	16.6	14.7	16.5	11.7	13.3	13.2	15.2
Adjective	7.0	6.3	6.5	9.1	9.1	6.9	10.5	12.0	10.5	10.7
Adverb	.001	1.5	3.1	3.2	2.6	2.3	4.7	4.7	5.6	8.4
Pronoun	17.8	8.1	9.9	11.8	13.6	11.2	11.2	8.8	9.9	11.1
Preposition	9.0	7.9	7.5	9.4	8.9	8.7	7.8	10.5	10.6	8.7
Conjunction	1.4	1.8	4.7	4.5	4.2	4.9	7.0	6.4	6.4	6.2
Article	17.4	15.9	15.0	14.3	13.7	15.5	12.4	10.0	11.9	8.9

TABLE IV

COMPARISON OF USAGE OF SELECTED PARTS OF SPEECH

		Number of times used by:	
Age	Part of Speech	Deaf	Hearing
7	Adverb	1	18
	Preposition	12	67
	Conjunction	18	38
9	Adverb	29	108
	Preposition	151	180
	Conjunction	34	163
11	Adverb	65	118
	Preposition	157	266
	Conjunction	98	162
13	Adverb	95	177
	Preposition	273	331
	Conjunction	131	199
15	Adverb	84	379
	Preposition	286	394
	Conjunction	133	281

ied, both groups were comparable; they demonstrated more nouns, followed by verbs, pronouns, and prepositions. Analysis of the data suggests certain differences in language usage that may be related to developing thought processes. At seven years, more than half (55.8 percent) of the deaf vocabulary consisted of nouns; the corresponding figure for the hearing was 38.3 percent. The higher usage of the concrete "naming level" was reflected throughout the age levels for the hearing impaired. Although the proportion decreases, the deaf consistently used more nouns than the hearing. For the hearing, the proportions of the various parts of speech remained constant throughout the age groupings; for the deaf, the use of prepositions was not attained until 9 years, while consistent use of conjunctions was not observed until 13 years, and only rudimentary use of adverbs was attained by age 15.

From these data conclusions may be drawn as to the development of mental processes on the part of the deaf; each of the areas in which the deaf show deficiency may be considered related to the development of abstract thought. Prepositions must be employed in order to record precise relationships, while conjunctions serve the purpose of unifying two or more thoughts and permits a relationship derived from discrete experiences to appear. Adverbial terms are employed to express qualifications and relationships. Such words are necessary for the expression of the abstract aspects of intelligence. The lack of adverbial usage appears related to the findings of consistent inferiority in reasoning ability.

A further limiation of the written thought processes may be observed in overuse of words. The 30 most frequently used words for each of the groups were tallied and compared; the data are presented in Table V. For the deaf at age seven, ten words made up almost 60 percent of the written product; 30 words represented 81.9 percent. For the hearing, the figures were 45.7 percent for the ten most frequently used words, and 68.9 percent for the thirty. At fifteen years of age, 30 words still accounted for more than half of the written words of the deaf. Because of their limited vocabulary, they must use the same word over and over, even though the word chosen may not be the choice to express correctly the desired concept.

Educators of the deaf have been aware of the difficulty of teaching verb tense to the hearing-impaired. Ability to use a verb

TABLE V

PERCENTAGE OF TOTAL WORDS ACCOUNTED FOR BY THE
FIRST 10, 20, AND 30 MOST FREQUENTLY USED

Age	Most frequent	Deaf	Hearing
7	10 words	59.2	54.8
	20 words	74.3	60.5
	30 words	81.9	68.9
9	10 words	44.9	34.8
	20 words	59.4	46.4
	30 words	67.3	53.9
11	10 words	40.9	30.5
	20 words	53.8	42.4
	30 words	61.8	49.5
13	10 words	35.7	32.6
	20 words	47.3	44.8
	30 words	55.2	50.8
15	10 words	38.5	26.1
	20 words	49.5	35.4
	30 words	56.5	40.7

in all its various forms is necessary if time and other referential relationships are to be established and maintained. The deaf child's lack of a time concept often has been noted and has served as a rationale for the inclusion of untimed tests in intellectual evaluation. Capacity to express action in terms of a past or future or a conditional even reflects the ability of the organism to detach itself from the present; the greater the ability to remove oneself from the here and now, the greater is the abstract mental function that can be assumed. To explore this concept further, the verbs of both the deaf and hearing were classified as to tense, and the usage was compared. The results as observed in Tables VI and VII were as expected. At seven years of age, both

TABLE VI

COMPARISON OF USE OF TENSES

	Deaf		Hearing	
Age	No. times used Present tense	No. times used Past tense	No. times used Present tense	No. times used Past tense
7	125	29	94	36
9	327	64	103	167
11	259	74	100	234
13	273	192	148	264
15	310	153	251	339

TABLE VII

COMPARISON OF THE USE OF COMPOUND VERBS

Age	Deaf No. times used	Hearing No. times used
7	—	31
9	108	102
11	46	80
13	38	101
15	69	203

the deaf and hearing were comparable in the greater use of the present tense; this finding was not unexpected, as children learning to read and write may not have been taught the various verb tenses in the printed form. Beginning at nine years of age, however, there was the consistent trend for the hearing to use the past more frequently than the present; for the deaf the trend was reversed. Even including the fifteen-year-olds, the deaf employed the present tense two to eight times more frequently than the past.

The overuse of the present tense may be considered another example of the immaturity of the language processes. A further example of this immaturity may be observed in the use of the compound verb form; in English, the compound verb serves to express tense, especially in the use of such concepts as the present progressive, the past perfect, the future perfect, conditional, and

TABLE VIII

COMPARISON OF VOCABULARIES USED EXCLUSIVELY
BY THE DEAF AND THE HEARING

Age Part of speech	Percentage of total vocabulary used exclusively by the deaf.					Percentage of total vocabulary used exclusively by the hearing.				
	7	9	11	13	15	7	9	11	13	15
Noun	70.7	40.8	48.1	51.5	51.1	58.1	64.4	46.8	55.1	70.6
Verb	50.0	38.7	66.9	54.8	58.6	75.0	80.7	73.8	75.5	79.8
Adjective	66.7	45.5	59.1	54.7	56.3	55.0	61.5	72.2	62.6	72.2
Adverb	——	27.8	55.2	30.1	34.3	100.0	75.0	64.9	64.6	79.5

the subjunctive. It appears that the complexity of the thought depends on how aptly the verb form fits what the writer has in mind. As noted in Table VII, the seven-year-old deaf did not have compound forms; at nine years, the groups were equal. This finding may be expressed by the fact that half of the deaf product consisted of the phrase "is playing." By eleven years, the hearing were using twice as many compounds; at thirteen, three times as many; and at fifteen, almost four times as many.

Apparently the deaf and the hearing approach the writing task differently as exemplified by the words they choose to express their thoughts. Considering just the use of the four parts of speech (see Table VIII) one has the impression that the two groups are using separate vocabularies as they write a story. At all age levels more than half the words written either by the deaf or hearing youngster were used exclusivly by their own group. The hearing children, however, made more use of words that were common to both groups. Preliminary evaluation of the noun material suggests that the deaf tend to use more words related to parts of the body or names of relatives. A hypothesis could be established that the deaf use these forms because of the exaggerated need for self-identification and to establish relationships. A more plausible hypothesis suggests that the deaf use the words that they know, and use them over and over. The words they know are derived more from what they have been taught than what they are able to pick up from conversations with peers, and these are what educators have felt that they should learn.

Discussion

It has been established that sensory deprivation as represented by profound deafness from early life has a significant effect on the development of mental processes. It has been shown that the lack of audition has lasting effects on such processes as memory and the use of abstractions. Further exploration is needed to determine whether the concreteness is a cause or a consequence of limited language development. The deaf child who has developed abstract reasoning beyond the limits of his language facility cannot express the ideas that he has, in turn further delimiting his verbal experience. Remediation must strike at the basis of the problem. Question may be raised as to the validity of training to develop specific mental processes, yet experience derived from work with those with learning disabilities has demonstrated that various aspects of memory can be improved, that proper selection of experience and vocabulary can raise the level of abstract behavior. If the language of the deaf could thereby be affected, a reciprocal development in mental processes would also appear.

References

Birch, Jack R., and J. W. Birch. 1957. "The Leiter International Performance Scale as an Aid to the Psychological Study of Deaf Children." *Am. Ann. Deaf*, **96**:503–511.

Blair, Frank. 1957. "A Study of the Visual Memory of Deaf and Hearing Children." *Am. Ann. Deaf*, **102**:254–263.

Bruner, J. S. 1964. "The Course of Cognitive Growth." *Am. Psychologist*, **19**:1–15.

Farrant, Roland. 1964. "The Intellective Abilities of Deaf and Hearing Children Compared by Factor-Analysis." *Am. Ann. Deaf*, **109**:305–306.

Furth, H. 1966. *Thinking without Language*. New York: The Free Press.

Gaeth, John. *Verbal and Nonverbal Learning in Children Including Those with Hearing Losses:* Co-operative Research Project No. 1001, Detroit: Wayne State University.

Gaeth, John. 1960. *Verbal Learning Among Children with Reduced Hearing Acuity*. Final Report of Project 289, U. S. Office of Educ., Submitted by Wayne State University Hearing Clinic.

Heider, Fritz., and Grace M. Heider. 1941. "Studies in the Psychology of the Deaf." *Psychol. Monog*. #242.

Luria, Aleksander. 1961. *The Role of Speech in the Regulation of Normal and Abnormal Behavior*. London: Pergammon.

Myklebust, Helmer R., Arthur I. Neyhus, and Ann Mullholland. "Guidance and Counseling for the Deaf." *Am. Ann. Deaf*, **107**:370–415.

Myklebust, Helmer. 1964. *The Psychology of Deafness* (Second Edition). New York: Grune & Stratton.

Neyhus, Arthur. 1962. "The Personality of Socially Well-Adjusted Deaf Adults as Revealed by Projective Test." Ph.D. Dissertation. Northwestern University.

Oleron, Pierre. 1953. "Conceptual Thinking of the Deaf." *Am. Ann. Deaf*, **38**:304–310.

Piaget, Jean. 1960. *Psychology of Intelligence*. Paterson, N. J.: Littlefield, Adams.

Pintner, Rudolph, Jon Eisenson, and M. Stanton. 1946. *The Psychology of the Physically Handicapped.* New York: F. S. Crofts.

Templin, M. C. 1950. *The Development of Reason in Children with Normal and Defective Hearing.* Minneapolis: U. of Minn. Press.

Vygotsky, Lev. 1962. *Thought and Language.* Cambridge, Mass.: The M.I.T. Press.

Wechsler, David. 1958. *The Measurement of Adult Intelligence.* Baltimore: Williams and Wilkins.

Werner, Heinz, and Donald Kaplan. 1963. *Symbol Formation: An Organismic Developmental Approach to Language and the Expression of Thought.* New York: Wiley.

Wright, Rogers. 1955. "The Abstract Reasoning of Deaf College Students." Ph.D. Dissertation. Northwestern University.

DISCUSSION: AUDIOLOGIC AND EDUCATIONAL TREATMENT AND RESEARCH

CHAPTERS in this section contain numerous references to the importance of the early detection of hearing-impaired children. The importance of early detection, of course, lies in being able to apply remedial measures—medical or surgical treatment if indicated, and habilitation procedures—at the earliest possible time. The whole emphasis in educational remediation is to minimize handicap, with the aim of producing adult citizens able to function effectively and productively in our society. Dr. Lowell stressed the three Ts—time, team, and technology—in relation to five steps in the psychoeducational management of the young deaf child. These five steps, you will recall, were awareness, acceptance, information, application, and teaching. You may remember that on the topic of application Dr. Lowell stated that only 6½ hours a day are available to the preschooler for the acquisition of language through the eyes. Although he did not stress this point, I am sure he would agree that it is also important to utilize the auditory channel as effectively as possible through all of the child's waking hours. The educational retardation of the deaf, a magnitude of some four to five years, was reported both by Dr. Lowell and by Drs. Neyhus and Myklebust. How best to close this educational gap? Dr. Lowell is too modest to say it, but more Tracy Clinics are obviously needed, with highly trained staffs and the latest technology to help parents put into application the information available about teaching language skills to preschool deaf children.

While Dr. Lowell's paper was concerned primarily with the management of the deaf child of preschool age and his parents, Dr. Connor stressed the education of school-age deaf children and pointed out the responsibilities of educators of the deaf, at the same time paying tribute to the many fine programs of training for preschool youngsters. Incidentally, I am sure that educators of the deaf agree that the deaf child who enters an educational program after he and his parents have received training in language development from such institutions as the Tracy Clinic and the Wilkerson Center is several steps ahead of the child who has not had the benefit of such training. Dr. Bender and Dr. Connor both mentioned that less than half of our preschool deaf population receive any specialized nursery school training on a daily basis. The need for the development of more such facilities is obvious.

For many decades the education of the deaf has followed traditional procedures, and the graduates of schools for the deaf have generally been graduated from high school with the equivalent of an eighth-grade education. As Dr. Lowell said, there has been discouragingly little improvement in the results achieved by educators of the deaf in the past forty-five years. Dr. Connor's chapter gives us reason to be optimistic that the picture may be changing as information from the fields of psychology, psychiatry, and linguistics is applied to improving techniques of instruction, both inside and outside the classroom. He is encouraged that within the framework of the Great Society the needs of the handicapped—including the deaf—are being recognized by our federal government, and funds are now available for research that we hope will result in improved methods in teaching the deaf. Funds are also available for universities to give professional preparation to increasing numbers of students who will become teachers of the deaf. There is hope now that the educational gap between the normal-hearing and the deaf high school graduate may be narrowed.

The chapters by Dr. Gaeth and by Drs. Neyhus and Myklebust reflect the increasing interest of universities in conducting research in methods of teaching the deaf. Educators have for years debated the relative importance of visual and auditory methods of teaching language to the deaf. Dr. Gaeth made reference to the work of the late Clarence Hudgins of Clarke School for the Deaf who was a pioneer in studying the effects of amplification in improving the language abilities of deaf children. In the *Journal of Speech and Hearing Disorders* (September 1953), Dr. Hudgins reported that his experimental group of deaf children who received auditory training with a specially designed group hearing aid of superior amplifying characteristics showed significant gains in both receptive and expressive language, thus arguing for a combined visual and auditory approach to teaching deaf children. In the May 1964 issue of *Asha*, Stewart, Pollock, and Downs reported on the advantages of what they called a "unisensory" method of teaching the deaf, suggesting that the auditory channel be used in teaching deaf children and that training in lipreading would impair the child's ability to learn language through the ear. Now Dr. Gaeth reports on some experiments that suggest the possibility that the visual channel of communications is superior to the auditory and that the combined audiovisual approach yields no better results than the visual approach alone. You will recall that Dr. Gaeth reported on studies of memorization, or rote learning, mostly with normal-hearing children, to see whether an audiovisual manner of presentation of material to be learned was more efficient than either an auditory or a visual method. His results indicated that the audiovisual approach, the "combined" approach, was no better than a single-modal approach, that is, either an auditory or a visual approach alone, whichever one was superior for the experiment at hand. He reported on two series of experiments. The first, before 1960, apparently utilized lists of paired simple words and compared learning rates by visual, auditory, and combined audiovisual presentations. Learning curves were obtained for normal-hearing and hearing-impaired children (grouped according to degrees of impairment). The experiment showed repeatedly that the combined presentation was not superior to the visual method with hard-of-hearing children, nor superior to either the visual or the auditory method with normal-hearing children. Because the experimenters believed their results might have been affected by the ease of the learning task, a second series of experiments was designed, using more difficult materials with gradations of "meaningfulness," and essentially the same results were obtained. While Dr. Gaeth did not present the results obtained with hearing-impaired children in the second series of experiments, he reported that their visual modality is so strong that it overrides the meaningfulness of the stimulus used.

Dr. Gaeth states that these data have important implications for the educational management of the hard-of-hearing and the deaf child. I am not sure on the basis of the data reported what conclusions can be drawn about the advantages of single-modal presentation of materials in a teaching situation, since Dr. Gaeth was reporting on the results of a highly structured experiment in the field of learning. I wish Dr. Gaeth had been more explicit in stating what the implications of his studies are for the educational management of the hearing-impaired child. Do the data argue for emphasizing the visual channel in the training of deaf children, or for giving more and better auditory training to improve the efficiency of the auditory channel? Perhaps the continuing investigation of these matters will yield the answer to this question.

In the chapter of Neyhus and Myklebust, the Myklebust Picture Story Test was administered to 800 deaf children at day and residential schools. From this group, 200 stories were selected and compared with an equal number obtained from a group of normal-hearing children matched by age, sex, and intelligence. The authors do not report the basis for their selection of only one out of four of the deaf sample. Data were presented from which conclusions were drawn concerning the language retardation of the deaf. In regard to the number of different words used by the subjects in their stories, I was struck by the similarities between the deaf and normal-hearing children through the age of 13, rather than by the differences. If the data are converted from tabular to graphic form, these similarities are more apparent. Vocabulary growth was a slowly accelerating curve for both groups, when I would have expected the normal-hearing group to show more rapid acceleration from one age category to the next. One wonders to what extent the story test actually reflects total vocabulary.

The authors conclude that the verbal deficiencies of the deaf may be related to the development of abstract thought; for example, they say, "The lack of adverbial usage appears related to the findings of consistent inferiority in reasoning ability." I am not sure that such conclusions are warranted on the basis of the data reported here, which are only a tabulation of word usage in a particular written-test situation. Admittedly it was not possible in this chapter to present all the data obtained in the national study of the psychology of deafness, and in the context of the total study such conclusions as reported here might well be considered appropriate.

EPILOGUE

A DOCTOR LOOKS AT «HAMLET»;
OR, MURDER MOST FOUL

The tragedy of *Hamlet, Prince of Denmark* was written by Shakespeare about 1599, and the world has been arguing about it ever since. In an introduction to Folio Society's edition of *Hamlet,* the actor Richard Burton writes (1954):

> It has been estimated that some 10,000 books, articles, and theses have been written on *Hamlet* which suggests that it is by far the most controversial play in the canon. It would also suggest that there can be very little to add.

Whilst agreeing that *Hamlet* is Shakespeare's most controversial play, I am venturing to add some new observations on the play. As an otologist I have always been intrigued by how Hamlet's father died. Pouring poison into the victim's ear is surely a unique method of murder, but how did the poison get from the ear into the system? And what was the poison used on Laertes' sword? Before I try to answer these questions let us consider briefly the scene of the action of the play and the leading seven characters, all of whom by the way came to a violent end, one before the play begins and the other six during the course of the play. The scene of action is Kronborg Castle, Elsinore, Denmark. The time is about the thirteenth century, and at that time Elsinore was the most important place in Denmark, being in the narrowest part of the sound giving access from the Baltic to the North Sea. The strongly fortified Elsinore could demand a toll from all ships that passed this point and these dues contributed handsomely to the Danish budget.

The play opens two months after the sudden and unexpected death of King Hamlet. The throne has been usurped by his brother Claudius who has also married the late King's widow. Hamlet, the late King's son, was distracted with grief at his beloved father's death and disgusted at the indecent haste with which his uncle and his mother had married. Thus we are faced with an efficient and worldly King, an attractive Queen, and a passionately grieving young Prince.

The principal characters are as follows:

The Ghost of King Hamlet

who it was given out died from being stung in the ear by a serpent. He plays a vital part in the play by revealing to his son, Prince Hamlet, on the platform before the castle of Kronborg during the night watch that

> The serpent that did sting
> thy father's life, now wears
> his crown,
> Thus was I, sleeping, by a
> brother's hand,
> of life, of crown, of queen
> at once dispatched.

Hamlet, Prince of Denmark

This unhappy, the "sweet prince" around whom the play revolves had to bear repeated shocks and emotional upheavals that might easily have unhinged a lesser man. Though it is suggested that he is a man of thirty, his emotional behavior is that of a much younger man and is essentially that of a rebellious youth against a stepfather who has ruined his family life.

Starting with the sudden death of his beloved father the King, his uncle usurps the throne and within a month has married his mother. Then Hamlet hears the dreadful truth from the ghost of his father. The ghost urges Hamlet,

> Let not the royal bed of Denmark be
> a couch for luxury and damned incest
> but howsoever thou pursuest this act,
> Taint not thy mind, nor let thy soul contrive
> Against thy mother aught; leave her to heaven.

Hamlet vows revenge referring to his mother and stepfather as

> O most pernicious woman.
> Oh villain, villain, smiling damned villain....

His essentially gentle nature regrets the role he is bound to play with,

> The time is out of joint; O cursed spite,
> That ever I was born to set it right.

Hamlet's emotions receive a further shock by the behavior of Ophelia whom he loves, but who now avoids him and will not answer his letters. Disillusioned by the behavior of his mother, he fears that his lovely Ophelia may have also fallen under the spell of his uncle. He enters her sewing chamber distraught and dishevelled.

> And with a look so piteous in purport,
> As if he had been loosed out of hell . . .

He gazes on her face for a while before leaving the room without a word. Later when they meet again Hamlet no doubt with his stepfather in mind urges her

> Get thee to a nunnery, Go, farewell.

When at the prompting of Hamlet a band of visiting players re-enacts the late King's murder, Claudius realizes that Hamlet knows the truth about his father's death. Queen Gertrude, fearing for Hamlet, asks him to visit her that same evening. Polonius the Chamberlain who brings the message from the Queen to Hamlet arranges with the King's contrivance to hide behind a curtain in the Queen's room during the meeting.

On his way to the Queen's closet, Hamlet comes upon King Claudius who is kneeling at prayer. Hamlet after a moment of indecision decides not to kill the King while he is in prayer.

The unfortunate Polonius as he hides in the Queen's closet is stabbed to death by Hamlet who thinks that the eavesdropper is the King.

The King decides that Hamlet must be got rid of and sends him on a journey to England with the message:

> The present death of Hamlet, Do it England.

Hamlet's ship is attacked by pirates two days out from Elsinore and he contrives to escape on to the pirate ship which bears him back to Denmark.

He arrives at Elsinore just in time for the funeral of poor Ophelia, who had lost her wits and drowned herself for love of Hamlet. Her brother Laertes, overcome with grief and passion at the death of his sister and father, both on account of Hamlet, is a ready and willing tool for the schemes of King Claudius against his rebellious stepson who knows the truth, who has escaped the first trap set by the King, and who must be eliminated without his mother or the people of Denmark, both of whom love the Prince, realizing what is happening.

King Claudius

ascended the throne of Denmark after the sudden death of his elder brother, King Hamlet. Within a month he had married his brother's widow and had taken a firm hold on the reins of power. Genial, efficient and sure of himself, he neatly put himself in the right in his opening speech to the court when he pointed out the need for a firm government after his brother's death with the threats from abroad, particularly Norway, and he commiserated with Hamlet's distress but pointed out that continued excess of sorrow for the death of a father was a little out of place. Efficient and bland, he earned the remark by Hamlet,

That one may smile, and smile and be a villain.

Until the revelation by the ghost of Hamlet's father, neither Hamlet, nor for that matter the audience, knew that Claudius had murdered his brother in order to usurp the throne and marry his widow.

After the players had enacted the murder, King Claudius realized that Hamlet knew what had happened and decided that Hamlet would have to go. This had to be carried out with circumspection because Hamlet was popular with the country and beloved of his mother. Kneeling at his confessional he admits his guilt:

O wretched state! O bosom, black as death.
O limed soul, that struggling to be free,
Art more engag'd.

Hamlet who witnesses this cannot bring himself to kill his stepfather at prayer, evades the English mission, and on his arrival back at Elsinore the King takes advantage of Laertes' anger against Hamlet, the man who killed his father and drove his sister to suicide, to enlist his help in the downfall of Hamlet. A duelling contest is proposed and Laertes suggests

And for that purpose I'll anoint my sword;
I bought an unction of a mountebank,
So mortal, that but dip a knife in it,
Where it draws blood, no cataplasm so rare,
... can save the thing from death,
that is but scratch'd withal.

The King to be doubly sure adds,

> As makes your bouts more violent to that end,
> And that he calls for drink; I'll have prepared him
> A chalice for the nonce; where on the sipping,
> If he by chance escape your venom'd stick,
> Our purpose may hold there.

Queen Gertrude,

wife of the late King Hamlet and mother of Prince Hamlet, married her late husband's brother within a month of his death. This double shock was almost too much for Prince Hamlet, the loss of a beloved father and his mother's marriage to his uncle—an uncle who had moreover usurped the throne led to Hamlet's outburst.

> Frailty thy name is woman. . . .
> He underlined the deed which so disgusted him.
> . . . married with mine uncle,
> My father's brother: but no more like my father,
> Than I to Hercules, within a month!

Though Shakespeare does not say so in so many words many feel that the Ghost of King Hamlet at his first meeting with Prince Hamlet suggests that there may have been an understanding between Claudius and Gertrude before King Hamlet died. The Ghost speaking of Claudius says

> Ay that incestuous, that adulterate beast
> With withcraft of his wits, with traitorous gifts
> . . . Won to his shameful lust
> The will of my most seeming virtuous Queen.

After the group of strolling players has enacted, at the instigation of Prince Hamlet, the late King's death, King Claudius with his new Queen and attendants leave the play abruptly and obviously offended. Soon afterwards the Queen sends Prince Hamlet a message through Polonius asking him to come to her room. Hamlet agrees and includes the following in a short soliloquy.

> I will speak daggers to her, but use none.

The unfortunate Polonius proposes to conceal himself in the Queen's closet and to report back to Claudius the result of her interview with Hamlet. As we know, Polonius is stabbed to death through the curtain by Hamlet who mistakes him for the King. He upbraids his mother who at first chides him with,

> *What have I done, that thou dare'st say thy tongue,*
> *In noise so rude against me?*

But nothing will stop Hamlet, so that in the end the Queen entreats:

> *O Hamlet, speak no more,*
> *Thou turn'st mine eyes into my very soul.*

And after another short but nasty description by Prince Hamlet of the King and Queen:

> *O speak to me no more,*
> *These words like daggers enter in mine ears,*
> *No more sweet Hamlet.*

But the most moving part of the closet scene is the return of the Ghost, not in armour this time but in night attire, his avowed purpose being to strengthen Hamlet's resolve, weakened perhaps by his mother's distress. To Hamlet's and the Ghost's dismay, the Queen sees and hears nothing and is confirmed in her fear of Hamlet's madness. The scene ends with a moving plea by Hamlet to the Queen not to return to King Claudius' bed.

Polonius

is chief councillor of the King, and as such has to obey his ruler and carry out his policies. He also has to try to keep the peace between the new King Claudius and the young Prince Hamlet, passionately grieving at the death of his father and outraged and disgusted at the hasty marriage of his mother to the man who has robbed him of his birthright, the throne. Naturally enough, Hamlet despises Polonius, the hunter with hare and runner with hounds, and affects to regard him as a silly and scheming old fool. Poor Polonius does his best but nothing seems to go right. By warning his daughter Ophelia against Hamlet he precipitates an estrangement between the two which ends tragically both for Ophelia and for Hamlet. In his eagerness to help his master the King and also to try and ascertain for himself the extent of and reason for Hamlet's wayward behavior, he plays eavesdropper with the King at a meeting between Hamlet and Ophelia. Hamlet, realizing he was being overheard, treats Ophelia as no better than a loose woman in the nunnery scene. In the closet scene between Hamlet and his mother the Queen, Polonius is accidentally stabbed to death by Hamlet through the curtain behind which he was hiding, mistaking him for the King. Hamlet's epitaph as he brings the body into a neighbouring room is

> ... *indeed this Councillor is now most still,*
> *Most secret, and most grave,*
> *Who was in life, a foolish prating knave.*

Laertes,

son of Polonius and brother of Ophelia, is a straightforward character whose problems and loyalties are simple and who acts as a foil to the much more complex Hamlet.

Laertes, who on the accession of the new King had returned from France for the coronation, now wishes to return there to complete his education. The King accedes to his request, though at the same audience declines for reasons of state to allow Hamlet to return to Wittenburg. Before leaving, Laertes warns his sister against the danger of an affair with Hamlet and is smartly reminded by his sister to behave circumspectly when he is in Paris.

On his return to Denmark, he is appalled to find his father killed, albeit accidentally, by Hamlet and his sister mad and soon drowned for the love of Hamlet. He needs but little encouragement by King Claudius to agree to a fencing contest with Hamlet and he himself suggests the poisoning of his own sword.

> *I will do 't,*
> *And for the purpose I'll anoint my sword:*
> *I bought an unction of a mountebank*
> *So mortal that but dip a knife in it,*
> *Where it draws blood no cataplasm so rare,*
> *Collected from all simples that have virtue,*
> *Under the moon, can save the thing from death.*

To make doubly sure, King Claudius replies,

> *When in your motion you are hot and dry*
> *As make your bouts more violent to that end*
> *And that he calls for drink: I'll have prepared for him*
> *A chalice for the nonce; whereon but sipping*
> *If he by chance escape your venom'd stick*
> *Our purpose may hold there.*

Ophelia

Our first glimpse of the lovely young Ophelia is in her father's home where first of all her brother Laertes warns her against the dangers of falling in love with a Prince. Then her father Polonius takes up the theme, and, finding that the Prince Hamlet and Ophelia have seen a lot of one another and have exchanged vows and gifts, forbids her to see Hamlet or even to answer his letters.

The effect of this upon the already distracted Hamlet brings things to a head so far as Polonius is concerned. For when Ophelia describes how Hamlet burst in upon her distraught and disarranged and held her at arms length staring at her intently but not saying a word, Polonius regards this as a sign of true love, and the King and Queen, when he tells them of it, are glad and hope that by encouraging the couple, Hamlet may come to his senses. Alas, the reason for Hamlet's mute scene with Ophelia is much more likely to be the effect of his mother's remarriage with Claudius and may be expressed by Hamlet's own phrase, "O frailty, thy name is woman"; and it may be that in his obsessive dislike of his uncle and stepfather, he fears that Ophelia's refusal to communicate with him was because of her attraction towards the lecherous King.

King Claudius and Polonius contrive a meeting between Ophelia and Hamlet which they can overhear. Ophelia offers back to Hamlet the gifts that he gave her and this provokes a lovers' quarrel made all the more bitter on Hamlet's part because he suspects they are being overheard, and this suspicion provokes his bitter nunnery speech which makes it clear to all who hear it that he is totally disillusioned by women and he ends with,

> Go to, I'll no more on't, it both made me mad
> I say, we will have no more marriages.
> Those that are married already, all but one shall live,
> The rest shall keep
> as they are. To a nunnery, go.

After Hamlet's exit the poor Ophelia remarks,

> And I of ladies most deject and wretched,
> That sucked the honey of his music vows;
> Now see that noble, most sovereign reason,
> Like sweet bells jangled out of time, and harsh.

At their next meeting—to witness the play—the unfortunate Ophelia is but a pawn in the contest between King Claudius and Hamlet. Hamlet chooses to sit by Ophelia in preference to his mother and then makes a few rather coarse jokes at Ophelia's expense, and for the rest of the scene Ophelia is used as a feed for the purpose of the play. Her next and last appearance is after Polonius' death at the hand of Hamlet. This has proved too much for her, and she has obviously lost her reason. The King and Queen note her state of mind, and her brother Laertes, newly returned from France, sees her and learns of his father's death remarking,

> O Heavens is't possible a young maid's wits
> Should be as mortal as an old man's life.

Ophelia drowns, presumably by her own hand, and at her funeral the priest points out,

> Her obsequies have been as far enlarged
> As we have warrantise, her death was doubtful.

The Queen says,

> Sweet to the sweet farewell
> I hop'd thou should'st have been my Hamlet's wife.

The Dueling Scene

Now we come to the final scene, the climax of the play.

King Claudius has wagered that in a duelling contest between Hamlet and Laertes, Laertes will not exceed Hamlet by more than three hits in a dozen passes. The weapons are foils and daggers, and as the whole court enters the stage the weapons are laid out together with flagons of wine. The two young men select their weapons, Laertes changes his for another, no doubt previously covered with poison, and just before the contest begins the King announces that if Hamlet scores the first or second hit he will drink to Hamlet's health and in the cup shall throw a pearl larger than any worn by previous Kings.

The contest begins. Hamlet scores a hit. The King drinks to Hamlet, drops the pearl, also covered with poison, and has it offered to Hamlet. Hamlet declines to drink at this moment, renews the contest, and scores another hit. During the pause, his mother Queen Gertrude wipes her son's face, and again Hamlet declines to drink at this moment; but in her excitement the Queen despite a warning cry from King Claudius takes a deep draught.

The contest is renewed with great vigor. Hamlet receives a wound on his arm. The foils are dropped in the scuffle and are exchanged so that Laertes is wounded by Hamlet, using the poisoned sword.

Laertes falls down, the Queen falls down dying saying,

> The drink, the drink I am poison'd.

Laertes tells Hamlet of the poisoned sword now in Hamlet's hand, whereupon Hamlet says,

> *The point envenomed too,*
> *Then venom to thy work.*

Whereupon he stabs the King and tries to make him drink from the cup saying,

> *Here thou incestuous murderous, damned Dane.*

The King dies and Hamlet who is prevented by his faithful friend Horatio from drinking from the poisoned cup says,

> *O I die Horatio;*
> *The potent poison quite o'ercomes my spirit,*
> *I cannot live to hear the news from England,*
> *But I do prophesy the election lights*
> *On Fortinbras.*

As Hamlet dies his friend Horatio says,

> *How cracks a noble heart;*
> *Good night sweet Prince*
> *And flights of Angels sing thee to thy rest.*

Then to tidy up the play, Fortinbras the young King of Norway and the English Ambassadors enter. The dreadful scene is explained. The English Ambassador reports the death of Rosencrantz and Gilderstern. Fortinbras takes charge saying,

> *Let four captains*
> *Bear Hamlet like a soldier to the stage.*

Thus all the principal characters are dead as the result of—
Two murders, King Hamlet and Prince Hamlet;
One suicide, Ophelia;
Three accidental homicides, Polonius, Queen Gertrude, Laertes;
One justifiable homicide, King Claudius.
And now let us consider in a little more detail the two murders. First that of King Hamlet and let his ghost tell the tale,

> *Sleeping within mine orchard*
> *My custom always in the afternoon,*
> *Upon my secure hour thy uncle stole,*
> *With juice of cursed hebona in a vial,*
> *And in the porches of mine ears did pour*
> *The leperous distilment.*

Now we want to know two things: What was the poison? How was it absorbed from the ear into the body?
The poison was almost certainly a vegetable alkaloid, and we

have a clue of what it was from elsewhere in the play. Reference is made to

> *Thou mixture of rank midnight weed collected.*

This surely must mean deadly nightshade, from which belladonna is derived. But how could it have been absorbed into the body from the outer-ear canal? Only if there was a larger perforation of the eardrum. Otitis media was very common in Shakespeare's day. Most families had at least one child who could not bathe because water ran into the throat from the ear. Shakespeare, ever a keen student of man, knew this, but who would know this better than a younger brother?

One final point: What made Shakespeare choose this unique way of introducing poison into the body? One explanation may be that about forty years earlier, just before Shakespeare was born, the youthful François II of France died, and it was put about, according to R. R. Simpson (1959), by a poisonous powder blown into his ear by his doctor, the famous Ambroïse Paré. Balzac's account of the king's death (like the ghost of Hamlet's father) offers a different reason (Coues, 1932). The youthful king caught a chill whilst on the River Loire. This went to his ear, which discharged and swelled up. Finally, intracranial infection supervened and Ambroïse Paré, the King's surgeon, was all in favor of opening the abcess from behind the ear. The King's consort, Mary Queen of France and, in her own right, of Scotland, was only too ready to accept Ambroïse Paré's advice. But her formidable mother-in-law, Catherine of Medici, forbade the operation and ordered Ambroïse Paré to inject the ear with fluid or with powder (Potiquet, 1893). The poor young King soon died, no doubt of an intracranial complication of otitis media, such as meningitis, a brain abscess, or lateral sinus thrombosis, and so the pathetic and youthful Mary lost the first of her two thrones.

This sad story no doubt came to Shakespeare's notice and may well have inspired him to employ this unusual method of introducing poison into the body. We must remember that at the time that Shakespeare wrote, otitis media was very common indeed, so that very few children grew to adult life without at least one perforated ear drum.

One of Shakespeare's favourite devices when dealing with royal personages was to make them appear as ordinary persons, and one way of doing this was to make them suffer from ordinary everyday disorders, such as, for instance, otitis media or its effects.

Another example of this may be seen in *Julius Caesar,* when we find (Act 1, scene 2) Caesar saying to Antony, "Come on my right hand, for this ear is deaf," and then a few lines later Brutus says to Casca and Cassius, speaking of Caesar, "Tis very like: he hath the falling sickness." This, I felt, pointed to Ménière's disease, rather than to epilepsy, as a cause of Caesar's falling sickness (Cawthorne 1958), and though there are several references in the Roman literature to Caesar's falling sickness, no one save Shakespeare mentions his deafness in one ear. Now what made him do that? Certainly nothing to do with stage business. I concluded that Shakespeare knew of the association between deafness in one ear and attacks of giddiness which lead to falling, and so as to give the human touch to one of his august heroes he introduced deafness in one ear. In so doing, Shakespeare preceded by 260 years Prosper Ménière's clinical description of 1861.

In the same way, Shakespeare must have known many people with a perforated ear drum, and being an astute clinical observer would have known, as all otologists and most sufferers from such a condition know, that fluid introduced into the ear by anyone with a perforated ear drum quickly finds its way into the throat. If the fluid were both warm and nonirritating to the ear and throat, then it might easily reach the throat and so be swallowed without arousing the victim.

And this, I believe, is how Hamlet's father was murdered. "Murder most foul" it certain was—and murder as ingenious as has ever been conceived.

Now let us consider the second murder by a poisoned sword of Prince Hamlet. The play was written in 1599, a little more than a century after Columbus landed in the West Indies. The Spaniards soon ventured to Central and South America, where they learned the deadly effect of the poisoned arrows of the natives. There is evidence that this poison was brought over to Europe in the middle of the sixteenth century, and of course we now know that the active ingredient of the poison on the arrows was curare. This I have no doubt was what Shakespeare had in mind when he had Laertes' sword tipped with curare. This is the only poison I know of which could have produced a fatal effect so quickly from a mere scratch.

Thus it is fair to say that poor King Hamlet was murdered by belladonna being poured into his ear. The poison reached his pharynx through a large perforation of the ear drum, it was swallowed and reached his stomach where it was absorbed into his system to produce its deadly effect. Prince Hamlet was murdered by Laertes' sword steeped in curare which had recently been brought to Europe from the newly discovered West Indies by Raleigh. By a curious turn of fate, the same poisoned sword accidentally killed Laertes and also the wretched King Claudius. The story of Hamlet was not a new one, but the genius of Shakespeare turned it into the greatest and the most controversial play that has ever been produced. It was written with the actor Richard Burbage in mind for the leading part. Its first performance was probably in the Blackfriars Playhouse, the relic of which is remembered by Playhouse Yard which now separates the offices of the *Times* from the building housing the Worshipful Society of Apothecaries, and it is interesting to recall that the earliest performances included Will Shakespeare himself as the ghost of King Hamlet.

References

Burton, R. 1954. "Introduction to the Tragedy of Hamlet Prince of Denmark." London: Folio Society.

"Balzac's Account of Ambroïse Paré and the Last Illness of Francis the Second."

Cawthorne, T. 1958. "Julius Caesar and the Falling Sickness. *Proc. Roy. Soc. Med.* **51**:27–30.

Coues, W. P. 1933. "Balzac's Account of Ambroïse Paré and the Last Illness of Francis the Second." *New England J. Med.* **208**:834.

Holmes, Martin. 1964. *The Guns of Elsinore.* London: Latti and Windus.

Potiquet, Albert. 1893. "La Maladie et la mort de François II Roi de." *Les végétationes adénoides dans l'histoire.* Paris: Rueff.

Simpson, R. R. 1959. *Shakespeare and Medicine.* Edinburg and London. p. 135.

Thomas, K. Bryn. 1964. *Curare, Its History and Usage.* London: Pitman Medical Publishing Guild.

Wilson, J. Dover, C. H. 1935. *What Happens in Hamlet.* Cambridge, England: Cambridge University Press.

INDEX

Sharla J. Haggerty